Chlamydia pneumoniae and Chronic Diseases

Springer-Verlag Berlin Heidelberg GmbH

Johanna L'age-Stehr (Ed.)

Chlamydia pneumoniae and Chronic Diseases

Proceedings of the State-of-the-Art Workshop
held at the Robert Koch-Institut Berlin
on 19 and 20 March 1999

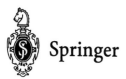 Springer

Editor:
DR. JOHANNA L'AGE-STEHR
Robert Koch-Institut
Nordufer 20
13353 Berlin

ISBN 978-3-540-41136-9

CIP data applied for
Chlamydia pneumoniae and chronic diseases : proceedings of the state-of-the-art workshop held at the Robert Koch-Institut Berlin on 19 and 20 March 1999 / Johanna L'age-Stehr (ed.). - Berlin ; Heidelberg ; New York ; Barcelona ; Hong Kong ; London ; Milan ; Paris ; Singapore ; Tokyo : Springer, 2000
ISBN 978-3-540-41136-9   ISBN 978-3-642-57195-4 (eBook)
DOI 10.1007/978-3-642-57195-4

This work is subject to copyright. All rights are reserved, whether the whole or part of the material is concerned, specifically the rights of translation, reprinting, reuse of illustrations, recitation, broadcasting, reproduction on microfilm or in any other way, and storage in data banks. Duplication of this publication or parts thereof is permitted only under the provisions of the German Copyright Law of September 9, 1965, in its current version, and permission for use must always be obtained from Springer-Verlag. Violations are liable for prosecution under the German Copyright Law.

© Springer-Verlag Berlin Heidelberg 2000
Originally published by Springer-Verlag Berlin Heidelberg New York in 2000

The use of general descriptive names, registered names, trademarks, etc. in this publication does not imply, even in the absence of a specific statement, that such names are exempt from the relevant protective laws and regulations and therefore free for general use.

Product liability: The publishers cannot guarantee the accuracy of any information about the application of operative techniques and medications contained in this book. In every individual case the user must check such information by consulting the relevant literature.

Editorial Assistance: Dr. Christiane Cordes
Copy-reader and Layout: Ursula Erikli
Image Analysis/Processing: Stefan Mertens
Typesetting: Camera ready by the editor
Cover design: *design & production GmbH*, Heidelberg
SPIN 10785123   18/3130/ag 5 4 3 2 1 0

Preface

J. L'age-Stehr

In March 1999 international experts from many fields gathered in Berlin for a State-of-the-Art Workshop on *Chlamydia pneumoniae* and chronic diseases. This workshop was the first of its kind initiated and organized by the Robert Koch-Institut.

The objectives of the workshop were to discuss and enhance interdisciplinary knowledge on the possible etiological role of *Chlamydia pneumoniae*, a widespread human respiratory infection, in the pathogenesis of chronic inflammatory diseases with major public health impact such as

- atherosclerosis,
- cardiovascular disease,
- adult-onset asthma bronchiale,
- chronic obstructive pulmonary disease,
- reactive arthritis,
- Morbus Alzheimer and
- Multiple Sclerosis.

An association of *Chlamydia pneumoniae* infections and atherosclerosis has been indicated by serological methods and by detection of the agent in vascular tissues. Major goals of this workshop were to identify current deficiencies in knowledge and research approaches, quality of methodologies used for detection of the infection, designs of epidemiological studies and to encourage prioritization of approaches in basic, applied and clinical research in a collaborative, multidisciplinary and multicenter effort.

Some of the experimental evidence put forward to the audience by the experts supported the hypothesis that recurrent or chronic persistent and reactivated *Chlamydia pneumoniae* infections may be risk factors in atherogenesis and the development of cardiovascular disease, in asthma bronchiale of adult onset and chronic obstructive pulmonary disease.

Evidence that these infections initiate, perpetuate or accelerate these major diseases when combined with other risk factors was vividly discussed as well as were the goals of future research. The possible involvement of *Chlamydia pneumoniae* in the pathogenesis of neurological diseases such as Morbus Alzheimer and Multiple Sclerosis met with considerable skepticism.

On the basis of current knowledge the following goals for future basic and applied research have been identified:

- encouragement and promotion of international multicenter, multidisciplinary collaborations of clinical and basic researchers for development and application of standardized noninvasive diagnostic tools for the detection of chronic *Chlamydia pneumoniae* infections,

- analysis of the influence of host genetics, classical identified risk factors and different agent–host interactions on susceptibility to chronic, recurrent or reactivated *Chlamydia pneumoniae* infections and the development of chronic diseases,
- search for surrogate diagnostic markers for chronic inflammation by *Chlamydia pneumoniae* infections to develop better diagnostic strategies that would identify subpopulations of patients at risk for cardiovascular diseases which would profit from antimicrobial therapy,
- promotion of more basic research on the natural history and pathogenicity of chronic, persistent and reactivated *Chlamydia pneumoniae* infections,
- inclusion of better standardized and expanded diagnostic strategies in design and monitoring of epidemiological cohort and case control studies,
- encouragement to develop better antimicrobial agents and therapeutic strategies and regimens (e.g. combinations of antibiotics) to increase treatment efficacy in subpopulations of chronic diseased patients with chronic, reactivated or remittent *Chlamydia pneumoniae* infections and use of more standardized diagnostic methodology to monitor efficacy of antimicrobial therapy in selected groups of patients.

All comments and questions in response to individual presentations have been enclosed in these proceedings to give the readers interested in the field of *Chlamydia pneumoniae* and chronic diseases a life-like picture of the often diverse opinions of the experts.

Introduction – *R. Kurth* 1

Chapter 1
Biology, Immunology and Pathology of *Chlamydia Pneumoniae* Infections

1.1 Pathogenic mechanisms of chronic *Chlamydia* infections

E. Straube, J. Rödel 3

1.2 Biology, immunology and persistence of *Chlamydia pneumoniae*: Links to chronic disease

G.I. Byrne and M.V. Kalayoglu 8
Chronic chlamydial diseases: *C. pneumoniae* and atherosclerosis 9
Chlamydial Hsp60 and the chronic disease process 10
Summary 11

1.3 Animal models for *Chlamydia pneumoniae* infection

M. Leinonen and P. Saikku 19
Monkey models for *C. pneumoniae* infection 19
Mouse models for *C. pneumoniae* infection 19
Rabbit model for *C. pneumoniae* infection 20
Animal models for *C. pneumoniae*-associated atherosclerosis 20
Conclusions 21

1.4 Molecular biology and serodiagnostics of *Chlamydia pneumoniae* – potential way to a vaccine

G. Christiansen, A.S. Madsen, T. Boesen, K. Hjernø, L. Daugaard, K. Knudsen, P. Mygind, S. Birkelund 25
Introduction 25
The GGAI gene family 25
Migration of GGAI proteins in SDS-PAGE 27
Antigenicity of GGAI proteins 27
Immunoblotting with human sera 28
Conclusion and considerations for future work 29

Chapter 2
Diagnosis of *Chlamydia pneumoniae* Infections

2.1 Direct detection of *Chlamydia pneumoniae* in atherosclerotic plaques

M. Maass 33
Introduction 33
Immunohistochemistry 35
PCR 35
Cell Culture 37
Conclusion 37

2.2 Detection of *Chlamydia pneumoniae* DNA in white blood cells
  J. Boman 42
2.3 Detection of *Chlamydia pneumoniae* in clinical specimens by PCR-EIA
  C.A. Jantos 48
2.4 State of the art in the diagnosis of acute and chronic *Chlamydia pneumoniae* infection
  M.R. Hammerschlag 52
  Culture of *C. pneumoniae* 52
  Detection of antibody to *C. pneumoniae* in serum 53

Chapter 3
Chronic Diseases Possibly Associated with *Chlamydia pneumoniae* Infections

3.1 Epidemiological data on respiratory tract infection with *Chlamydia pneumoniae* and clinical complications
  J. Boman 63
3.2 Role of *C. pneumoniae* in severe asthma and COPD: Epidemiology and treatment
  R. Cosentini, F. Blasi 68
  Asthma 68
  Chronic bronchitis 69
3.3.1 *Chlamydia pneumoniae* in atherosclerosis
  P. Saikku 73
  Introduction 73
  Epidemiological and seroepidemiological findings 73
  Histopathological studies 74
  Intervention trials 74
  Possible pathogenetic mechanisms by which an infection could affect the development of atherosclerosis and coronary heart disease. 75
  Conclusions 76
3.3.2 Prevalence of *Chlamydia pneumoniae* in human coronary plaques with acute coronary syndrome
  G. Bauriedel, U. Welsch and B. Lüderitz 84
  Introduction 84
  Patients and methods 85
  Results 85
3.3.3 Chlamydial lipopolysaccharide and atherosclerosis
  H. Brade 91
3.3.4 Clinical trial designs to study antibiotic intervention in atherosclerosis
  M. Dunne 97

3.3.5 Why antibiotics against *Chlamydia pneumoniae* for treatment of atherosclerotic disease could fail
  J.M. Ossewaarde 103
3.3.6 Atherosclerosis: Why the search for a causative infectious agent is not warranted
  S. Bhakdi 108
3.4 Chlamydia infections and arthritis
  J. Sieper 112
3.5 *Chlamydia pneumoniae*, APOE genotype, and Alzheimer's disease
  A.P. Hudson, H.C. Gérard, J.A. Whittum-Hudson, D.M. Appelt, B.J. Balin 121
  Alzheimer's disease 121
  APOE allele types and Alzheimer's disease 122
  Pathogenesis and epidemiology of *Chlamydia pneumoniae* 122
  Chlamydia pneumoniae DNA in the Alzheimer's brain 123
  Ultrastructural analysis of *Chlamydia pneumoniae* in the Alzheimer's brain 124
  Culture of *Chlamydia pneumoniae* from Alzheimer's brain tissue 126
  Immunohistochemical analyses 126
  Chlamydia pneumoniae infection and *APOE* allele types 128
  Future research directions 128
3.6 Association of *Chlamydia pneumoniae* with Multiple Sclerosis: Protocol for detection of *C. pneumoniae* in the CSF and summary of preliminary results
  C.W. Stratton, S. Sriram, S. Yao, A. Tharp, L. Ding, J.D. Bannan, W.M. Mitchell 137
  Introduction 137
  Materials and methods 137
  Results 143
  Discussion 148

Chapter 4
Epidemiology and Public Health Impacts of *Chlamydia pneumoniae* Infections

4.1 Trends and variations of chronic diseases in populations – Can infectious agents help to solve the puzzles?
  H.W. Hense 153

4.2 The epidemiology of *Chlamydia pneumoniae* versus the epidemiology of potential Chlamydial diseases (Atherosclerosis, Multiple Sclerosis, M. Alzheimer)

W. Stille, C. Stephan, M. Madeo, E. Bauer-Krylov 163
Epidemiology of *Chlamydia pneumoniae* 163
Seroepidemiology 163
Epidemiology of Multiple Sclerosis 167
Epidemiology of Alzheimer's Disease 168
Conclusion 168

4.3 The high male mortality of coronary heart diseases can be explained as a result of chronic infection

E. Bauer-Krylov, W. Stille 171

4.4 The *Spandauer Gesundheitstest* – Retrospective cohort study on *Chlamydia pneumoniae* infections and cardiovascular disease – A study concept

T. Ziese 178
Introduction 178
Study goals 178
Study outline 178

4.5 Public health impact of atherosclerosis and *Chlamydia pneumoniae* infections – What do we know and what to expect from future research

J.M. Ossewaarde 184
Introduction 184
Epidemiology of cardiovascular diseases in the Netherlands 184
Epidemiology of *Chlamydia pneumoniae* infections 185
Respiratory tract infections as a risk factor for cardiovascular disease 186
Association of *C. pneumoniae* infections and cardiovascular diseases 186
Public health consequences 187
Conclusions 187

Chapter 5
Final Discussion: Pro and Contra the Role of *Chlamydia pneumoniae* in Chronic Diseases 193

Presenting participants

Elisabeth Bauer-Krylov
Klinikum der J.W. Goethe-Universität
Theodor-Stern-Kai 7
D-60596 Frankfurt
Tel.:   +49-(0)-69-6301-5452
Fax: +49-(0)-69-6301-6378

Prof. Dr. Gerhard Bauriedel
Med. Universitätsklinik
Kardiologie/Pneumologie
Sigmund-Freud-Str.25
D-53105 Bonn
Tel.:   +49-(0)-228-287-6670
Fax: +49-(0)-228-287-4323
E-mail: g.bauriedel@gmx.de

Prof. Dr. Sucharit Bhakdi
Institut f. Med. Mikrobiologie u. Hygiene
Hochhaus am Augustusplatz
D-55101 Mainz
Tel.:   +49-(0)-6131-17-7341
Fax: +49-(0)-6131-39-2359
E-mail: makowiez@mail.uni-mainz.de

Dr. Jens Boman
University Hospital of Umeå
Dept. of Clinical Virology
S-901 85 Umeå
Sweden
Tel.:   +46-90-7851304
Fax: +46-90-129905
E-mail: jens.boman@climi.umu.se

Prof. Dr. med. Helmut Brade
Forschungszentrum Borstel
Med. und Biochem. Mikrobiologie
Parkallee 22
D-23845 Borstel
Tel.:   +49-(0)-4537-188-474
Fax: +49-(0)-4537-188-419
E-mail: hbrade@fz-borstel.de

Dr. Gerald I. Byrne
Dept. Med. Microbiology & Immunology
University of Wisconsin-Madison
1300 University Ave.
Madison, WI 53706-1532
USA
Tel.:   +1-608-263-2494
Fax: +1-608-262-8418
E-mail: gibyrne@facstaff.wisc.edu

Dr. Gunna Christiansen
Dept. Med. Microbiol. and Immunology
The Bartholin Building
University of Aarhus
DK-8000 Aarhus C
Denmark
Tel.:   +45-89-4217-49
Fax: +45-86-1961-28
E-mail: gunna@medmicro.au.dk

Dr. Roberto Cosentini
Institute of Respiratory Diseases
University of Milan, Pad. LITTA
Policlinico, Via F. Sforza, 35
I-20122 Milano
Italy
Tel.:   +39-02-5503-3614/-3602
Fax: +39-02-5519-0332
E-mail: medurg3@polic.cilea

Dr. Michael W. Dunne
Pfizer Inc.
Building 260 Room 1606
Eastern Point Road
Groton, CT 06340-8030
USA
Tel.:   +1-860-441-3739
Fax: +1-860-441-5702
E-mail: michael.w.dunne@
   groton.pfizer.com

Prof. Dr. Hermann Haller
Franz-Volhard-Klinik am
Max-Delbrück-Centrum für Mol. Medizin
Wiltbergstr. 50
D-13125 Berlin
Tel.: +49-(0)-30-9417-2203
Fax: +49-(0)-30-9417-2206

Prof. Dr. Margaret Hammerschlag
Department of Pediatrics, SUNY Health
Science Center at Brooklyn
New York, NY 11203
USA
Tel.: +1-718-245-4075
Fax: +1-718-245-2118
E-mail: MHammerschlag@POL.NET

Prof. Dr. Hans-Werner Hense
Institut für Epidemiologie und
Sozialmedizin der Wilhelms-Universität
Domagkstr. 3
D-48129 Münster
Tel.: +49-(0)-251-83-55399
Fax: +49-(0)-251-83-55300
E-mail: HENSE@UNI-MUENSTER.DE

Dr. Alan Hudson
Dept. of Immunology and Microbiology
Wayne State University
School of Medicine
Gordon H. Scott Hall
540 East Canfield Avenue
Detroit, MI 48201
USA
Tel.: +1-313-993-6641
Fax: +1-313-577-1355
E-mail: ahudson@med.wayne.edu

PD Dr. Christian A. Jantos
Institut für Medizinische Mikrobiologie
Klinikum der Justus-Liebig-Universität
Frankfurter Str. 107
D-35392 Giessen
Tel.: +49-(0)-641-99-41265
Fax: +49-(0)-641-99-41259
E-mail: Christian.Jantos@mikrobio.
med.uni-giessen.de

Prof. Dr. Reinhard Kurth
Direktor Robert Koch-Institut
Nordufer 20
D-13353 Berlin
Tel.: +49-(0)-30-4547-2000
Fax: +49-(0)-30-4547-2610
E-mail: haselbachg@rki.de

Dr. Johanna L'age-Stehr
Robert Koch-Institut
Nordufer 20
D-13353 Berlin
Tel.: +49-(0)-30-4547-2244
Fax: +49-(0)-30-4547-2604
E-mail: lage-stehrj@rki.de

Dr. Maija Leinonen
National Public Health Institute
Department in Oulu
Box 310
Fin-90101 Oulu
Finland
Tel.: +358-8-537-6235
Fax: +358-8-537-6251
E-mail: maija.leinonen@ktl.fi

PD Dr. med. Matthias Maass
Medizinische Universität zu Lübeck
Institut für Med. Mikrobiologie
Ratzeburger Allee 160
D-23538 Lübeck
Tel.: +49-(0)-451-500-2822
Fax: +49-(0)-451-500-2808
E-mail: maass@hygiene.mu-luebeck.de

Prof. Dr. Reinhard Marre
Ärztlicher Direktor
Abt. Med. Mikrobiologie und Hygiene
Inst. f. Mikrobiol. und Immunologie
Robert-Koch-Str. 8
D-89081 Ulm
Tel.:　+49-(0)-731-5024-600
Fax:　+49-(0)-731-5024-619
E-mail: reinhard.marre@medizin.uni-ulm.de

Dr. Jacobus M. Ossewaarde
Research Lab. for Infectious Diseases
National Institute for Public Health and the Environment
Antonie van Leeuwenhoeklaan 9
NL-3721 MA Bilthoven
Niederlande
Tel.:　+31-30-274-3942
Fax:　+31-30-274-4449
E-mail: JM.Ossewaarde@rivm.nl

Prof. Dr. Pekka Saikku
National Public Health Institute
Department in Oulu
Box 310
Fin-90101 Oulu
Finland
Tel.:　+358-8-537-6231/-6227
Fax:　+358-8-537-6222
E-mail: pekka.saikku@ktl.fi

Prof. Dr. Joachim Sieper
Univ.-klinikum Benjamin Franklin
Med. Klinik IV
Hindenburgdamm 30
D-12200 Berlin
Tel.:　+49-(0)-30-8445-4547
E-mail: hjsieper@zedat.fu-berlin.de

Prof. Dr. Wolfgang Stille
Klinikum der J.W. Goethe-Universität
Medizinische Klinik III
Theodor-Stern-Kai 7
D-60596 Frankfurt
Tel.:　+49-(0)-69-6301-5452/-6344
Fax:　+49-(0)-69-6301-6378

Prof. Dr. Charles W. Stratton
Vanderbilt University
Medical Center
2201 Capers Av.
Nashville, TN 37212, USA
Tel.:　+1-615-3439063
E-mail: Charles.Stratton@mcmail.vanderbilt.edu

Prof. Dr. Eberhard Straube
Institut f. Medizinische Mikrobiologie
am Klinikum der FSU Jena
Semmelweisstr. 4
D-07740 Jena
Tel.:　+49-(0)-3641-933-106
Fax:　+49-(0)-3641-933-474
E-mail: STRAUBE.BACH.RES.BACH.UKJ@BACH.MED.UNI-JENA.DE

Dr. Thomas Ziese
Robert Koch-Institut
General-Pape-Str.62-66
D-12101 Berlin
Tel:　+49-(0)-30-4547-3306
Fax:　+49-(0)-30-4547-3513
E-mail: zieset@rki.de

Additional participants

Prof. Dr. Bernd Appel
Robert Koch-Institut
Nordufer 20
D-13353 Berlin

Dr. Karsten Becker
Universität Münster
Institut für Med. Mikrobiologie
Domagkstr. 10
D-48149 Münster

Dr. Bärbel-Maria Bellach
Robert Koch-Institut
General-Pape-Str. 62–66
D-12101 Berlin

Lilo Berg
Berliner Zeitung
Karl-Liebknecht-Str.29
D-10178 Berlin

Dr. Berger
Franz-Volhard-Klinik
Max-Delbrück-Centrum f. Mol. Med.
Wiltbergstr. 50
D-13125 Berlin

Prof. Dr. Svend Birkelund
Dept. of Medical Microbiology and Immunology
The Bartholin Building
University of Aarhus
DK-8000 Aarhus C

Prof. Dr. Reinhard Burger
Robert Koch-Institut
Nordufer 20
D-13353 Berlin

Dr. Stephanie Czaika
Der Tagesspiegel
Potsdamer Str. 77-87
D-10785 Berlin

Dr. Essig
Abt. f. Med. Mikrobiologie u. Hygiene
Universität Ulm
D-89077 Ulm

Dr. Christian Gerischer
Humboldt-Krankenhaus
Am Nordgraben 2
D-13509 Berlin

Dr. med. J. Gieffers
Medizinische Universität zu Lübeck
Institut für Medizinische Mikrobiologie
Ratzeburger Allee 160
D-23538 Lübeck

Dr. Wolfgang Haist
I. Innere Abteilung
Krankenhaus Moabit
Turmstr. 21
10559 Berlin

Wiebke Hellenbrand
Robert Koch-Institut
Nordufer 20
D-13353 Berlin

Dr. Judith Whittum-Hudson
Dept. of Immunol. Microbiology
Wayne State University
School of Medicine
Gordon H. Scoot Hall
540 East Canfield Avenue
Detroit, MI 48201, U.S.A.

Dr. Gabriele Hundsdörfer
Bundesministerium für Gesundheit
Ref. 307
D-53127 Bonn

Prof. Dr. S.E. Kaufmann
Max-Planck-Inst. für Infektionsbiologie
Monbijoustr.2
D-10117 Berlin

Dr. med. St. Kempinski
Osthofener Weg 18
D-14129 Berlin

Dr. Andreas Klos
Med. Mikrobiologie
Med. Hochschule Hannover
Carl-Neuberg-Str. 1
D-30623 Hannover

A.C. Klucken
Charité – Humboldt-Universität
Med. Klinik II / Infektiologie
Augustenburger Platz 1
D-13353 Berlin

Klaus Koch
Süddeutsche Zeitung
Sandanger Str.8
D-80331 München

Frau Dr. Korfmann
Bayer AG
Business Group Pharma
D-42096 Wuppertal

M. Krüll
Charité – Humboldt-Universität
Med. Klinik II / Infektiologie
Augustenburger Platz 1
D-13353 Berlin

Prof. Dr. med. J. Kunz
Klinikum Ernst von Bergmann
Charlottenstr. 72
D-14467 Potsdam

Prof. Dr. med. Manfred L'age
II. Innere Abteilung
Auguste-Viktoria-Krankenhaus
Rubensstr. 125
D-12157 Berlin

Dr. Astrid Lewin
Robert Koch-Institut
Nordufer 20
D-13353 Berlin

Mazur Lüdger
Humboldt-Krankenhaus
Am Nordgraben 2
D-13509 Berlin

Dr. Ulrich Marcus
Robert Koch-Institut
Nordufer 20
D-13353 Berlin

Dr. May
Deutsches Herzzentrum München
Email: May@DHM.MHN.de

Dr. Klaus Melchert
Byk Gulden – Abt. FB 3
Lomberg Chem. Fabrik GmbH
Byk Gulden Str.2
D-78467 Konstanz

Dr. Inge Mühldorfer
Byk Gulden – Abt. FB 3
Lomberg Chem. Fabrik GmbH
Byk Gulden Str.2
D-78467 Konstanz

Edgar Muschketat
Robert Koch-Institut
Nordufer 20
D-13353 Berlin

PD Dr. Dieter Naumann
Robert Koch-Institut
Nordufer 20
D-13353 Berlin

Prof. Dr. Franz-Josef Neumann
Deutsches Herzzentrum und
1. Med. Klinik der TU
Lazarettstr. 36
D-80636 München

Prof. Dr. Georg Pauli
Robert Koch-Institut
Nordufer 20
D-13353 Berlin

Dr. Stefan Postius
Byk Gulden – Abt. FB 1
Lomberg Chem. Fabrik GmbH
Byk Gulden Str. 2
D-78467 Konstanz

Andrea Sommer
Hoechst Marion Roussel
Deutschland GmbH
Königsteiner Str. 10
D-65812 Bad Soden

Dr. Hartmut Steinrück
Robert Koch-Institut
Nordufer 20
D-13353 Berlin

Dr. Christian Stephan
Klinikum der J.W. Goethe-Universität
Theodor-Stern-Kai 7
D-60596 Frankfurt

Dr. Eckhard Strauch
Robert Koch-Institut
Nordufer 20
D-13353 Berlin

Dr. Sebastian Strigl MD
Division of Ped. Infectious Diseases
Department of Pediatrics
State University of New York
450 Clarkson Ave Box 49
Brooklyn NY 11203, U.S.A.

Dr. Kathrin Tintelnot
Robert Koch-Institut
Nordufer 20
D-13353 Berlin

Dr. Wolfgang Vettermann
Robert Koch-Institut
Nordufer 20
D-13353 Berlin

Dr. Edgar Werner
Robert Koch-Institut
General-Pape-Str. 62–66
D-12101 Berlin

Introduction

R. Kurth

Dear colleagues, I would very much like to welcome all of you to this special non-public state-of-the-art workshop about *Chlamydia pneumoniae and chronic diseases*.

I am very pleased that we were successful in assembling such an expert audience to exchange ideas and standpoints about diagnosis, treatment and prevention of Chlamydia infections and their possible relevance for the development of certain chronic diseases.

Why is the Robert Koch-Institut inviting to such a workshop? We are not working experimentally with Chlamydia. The Robert Koch-Institut as it stands today is no longer comparable to the one that existed before 1994. In 1994 – some of you may recall – the Federal Health Office, the *Bundesgesundheitsamt*, was dissolved and the old Robert Koch-Institut was united with the Institute for Social Medicine and Epidemiology. In addition, the AIDS-Center of the Federal Health Office was integrated. In recent years we have undergone not only a considerable restructuring but have also developed a new definition of who we are, what we are doing and what we should be doing in the future. And as a result we can really say that the Robert Koch-Institut is the Federal Health Institute engaged in applied – in part also in basic – research and in epidemiology. One of our tasks is the observation, prevention, and research of those diseases that have a high public impact or are of particular medical relevance. Coronary diseases certainly belong to this category.

As you all know, there is a controversial discussion – or has been a controversial discussion at least – about the role of chronic infections and disease development. We all remember the fascinating example of *Helicobacter pylori* infections in human diseases of the stomach. Obviously, we may have a second field here where a chronic bacterial infection may lead to various chronic diseases. And it is very timely that we hold the workshop this March 1999, especially as in the last few weeks and months additional data were published that suggest *in toto* an association between chronic Chlamydia infection and the development of diseases of the lung, of the arteries, and of the heart. In particular I am referring to the overview or retrospective study in *JAMA* in February '99 about the benefits of antibiotic treatment for the prevention of myocardial infarction.

Another point to be discussed is certainly the antigenic mimicry that has recently been described in a paper in *Science*, suggesting that outer membrane proteins of Chlamydia may lead to the induction of antibodies that cross-react with certain heart muscle proteins, including alpha myosin.

What are the aims of the workshop? Ideally, to obtain some answers from you as the leading international experts in the research on Chlamydia, to experience a state-of-the-art discussion, to review whether there is an association between *Chlamydia pneumoniae* infection and chronic diseases. It would also be important to identify deficits in research. In case there is an association or even causal relationship between Chlamydia infection and myocardial diseases or infarction, we should not try to develop prevention strategies that are based on the chronic use of antibiotics, because obviously we already have plenty of problems with antibiotic resistance. Instead, I believe, we ought to join those who have already started to think about the development of a vaccine against Chlamydia infections.

In summary, this infection has a very high visibility, a high prevalence in our population and, therefore, represents a significant public health problem. I hope that we will also have a very lively pro and con discussion tomorrow at the round table about the interpretation of data that may or may not suggest an association between infection and chronic disease development.

In that sense I hope we'll have a very fruitful, successful workshop.

Chapter 1
Biology, Immunology and Pathology of *Chlamydia pneumoniae* Infections

1.1
Pathogenic mechanisms of chronic *Chlamydia* infections

E. Straube, J. Rödel

Chlamydiae are obligate intracellular bacteria. The genus *Chlamydia* consists of the species *C. trachomatis*, *C. psittaci*, mostly pathogenic for animals, but with some human pathogenic strains, *C. pneumoniae*, and *C. pecorum*, pathogenic for cows and pigs. Recently, a bacterium called "Simkania Z" was related to *Chlamydia* on the 16 S rRNA level. *C. trachomatis* is divided into the serotypes A, B, and C, responsible for trachoma, the serotypes D–K, which cause common sexually transmitted infections of the genital mucous membranes, and the serotypes L1, L2, and L3, responsible for the lymphogranuloma venereum. *C. pneumoniae* is not divided into serotypes so far. It causes respiratory infections, chronic juvenile arthritis and is discussed in relation to the pathogenesis of intrinsic asthma and atherosclerosis.

Chlamydiae have a complicated biphasic life cycle consisting of an extracellular and an intracellular phase. The extracellular elementary bodies (EB) are the infectious form of this bacteria which have only minimal metabolic activity. These EB express outer membrane proteins on the surface that are necessary for an intimate adherence to so far not identified receptors on the host cell. The most predominant outer membrane protein of *C. trachomatis* is the major outer membrane protein (MOMP) with a N-linked high mannose type oligosaccharide moiety involved in adhesion and infectivity [12]. In *C. pneumoniae* the most immunodominant outer membrane proteins are Omp4 and Omp5 (97–99 kDa) as it could be shown in experimentally infected mice [11]. α-D-mannose and N-acetyl-D-galactosamine were found as inhibitors of the adhesion of *C. trachomatis* on synovial cells [3, 4]. Heparan sulfate and other sulfated polyanions were also identified as inhibitors of the infection of epithelial cells by *C. trachomatis* [10, 17].

The intimate adherence of the EB leads to their internalization by the host cell and to formation of an intracellular inclusion body. This process is accompanied by an increased phosphorylation of tyrosine-rich proteins in the host cell wall and cytosole, indicating a receptor-dependent signal transduction.. Proteins involved are those of 69/71 kDa, 75/85 kDa, and 100 kDa [5, 6, 9]. In *C. pneumoniae* infected HeLa cells the phosphorylation of tyrosine-rich receptor proteins could be observed only to a lower extent [7].

The process of adherence and internalization can be thought to be influenced by antibodies against the most immunodominant surface antigens of EB which are different in *Chlamydia trachomatis* and *Chlamydia pneumoniae*, the two most common species causing infections in man. The intracellular aggregation of internalized *C. trachomatis* EB followed by the formation of a single inclusion body in the host cell depends on the concentration of free intracellular Ca^{2+} and F-actin indicating the involvement of the signaling pathway network of the host cell [13]. In contrast to *C. trachomatis*, strains of *C. pneumoniae* can form multiple inclusion bodies within the host cell and do not utilize the cell microtubule network [7]. After internalization chlamydial cells multiply and form inclusion bodies containing up to 10^4 reticulate bodies (RB), cells with high metabolic activity and susceptibility to a wide range of antibiotics.

Chlamydia avoid the fusion of the inclusion bodies with lysosomal compartments in order to persist and replicate within the host cell. Proteins involved in this process are well known in *C. psittaci*, encoded in IncA, IncB, and IncC [1, 2]. Recently a homologous IncA protein was found in *C. trachomatis* [1].

Despite the high number of bacteria inside the inclusion bodies, the *Chlamydia trachomatis*-infected cell becomes less apoptotic as should be expected, compared with infections caused by other bacteria. There is evidence that *Chlamydia trachomatis* interferes with the apoptotic mechanism of infected host cells which are stimulated for apoptosis with staurosporin, etoposide, TNF-α, Fas antibodies, or granzyme B/perforin treatment. It could be shown that *Chlamydia* inhibits the downstream caspase 3 and the poly-(ADP-ribose)-polymerase and blocks the release of mitochondrial cytochrom C [8]. The inhibition of apoptosis could support a persistent infection with *Chlamydia*.

Attachment and internalization of *Chlamydia* upregulate the production of several cytokines by the infected cell (Figure 1). The cytokine network induced by *Chlamydia*-infected host cells and by subsequently activated macrophages and lymphocytes consists of factors which arrest the intracellular growth of the bacteria and inhibit the formation of regular EB. This could be shown with cytokines of the interferon family and with TNF-α [15]. In IFN-γ-treated fibroblasts *Chlamydia trachomatis* is suppressed in the expression of major outer membrane protein (MOMP), but enhanced in the expression of heat shock protein (HSP 60).

IFN-γ induces the expression of HLA class II molecules not only in macrophages, but also in non professional phagocytes. In *Chlamydia*-infected cultures of fibroblasts this mechanism is suppressed [14]. This may lead to an insufficient presentation of chlamydial antigens by these cells. Additionally, the infection of synovial cells with *C. trachomatis* upregulates the expression of interferon regulator factor 1 (IFR1). IFR1 can induce the expression of IFN-beta on one hand and on the other hand it upregulates the indoleamine 2,3-dioxygenase followed by a depletion of intracellular tryptophan. This leads to an inhibition of chlamydial growth within the inclusion body [16].

Thus, the intracellular growth, the impaired fusion of the inclusion bodies with lysosomal compartments, the inhibition of apoptosis, the delayed presentation of chlamydial antigens, and the inhibition of the growth and maturation of the reticulate bodies under the influence of the cytokine network in an infected tissue are mechanisms that may support a persistent infection with *Chlamydia*.

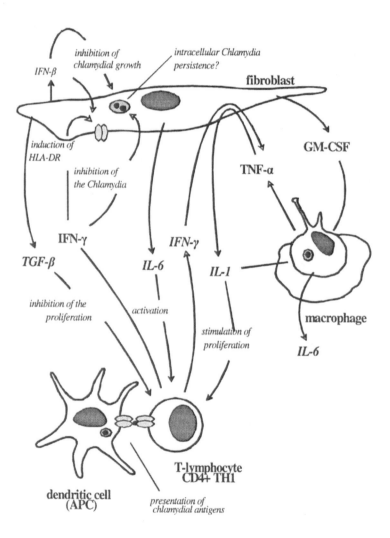

Figure 1. Model of the induction of cytokines in synovial cells after infection with *Chlamydia trachomatis* (from ref. [14]).

References

1. Bannantine JP, Stamm WE, Suchland RJ, Rockey DD (1998) *Chlamydia trachomatis* IncA is localized to the inclusion membrane and is recognized by antisera from infected humans and primates. Infect Immun 66: 6017–6021
2. Bannantine JP, Rockey DD, Hackstadt T (1998) Tandem genes of Chlamydia psittaci that encode proteins localized to the inclusion membrane. Mol Microbiol 5: 1017–1026
3. Berlau J, Ziemer A, Groh A, Straube E (1997) Influence of lectins on the infectivity of elementary bodies of *Chlamydia trachomatis* D IC CAL 8 by Synovial Cells. Eur J Clin Microbiol Infect Dis 16: 701–703
4. Berlau, J, Junker U, Groh A, Straube E (1998) In situ hybridization and use of direct fluorescence antibodies for detection of *Chlamydia trachomatis* in synovial tissue from patients with reactive arthritis. J Clin Pathol 51: 803–806
5. Birkelund S, Bini L, Pallini V, Sanchez-Campillo M, Liberatori S, Clausen JD, Ostergaard S, Holm A, Christiansen G (1994) Characterization of *Chlamydia trachomatis* l2-induced tyrosine-phosphorylated HeLa cell proteins by two-dimensional gel electrophoresis. Electrophoresis 18: 563–567
6. Birkelund S, Johnsen H, Christiansen G (1997) *Chlamydia trachomatis* serovar L2 induces protein tyrosine phosphorylation during uptake by HeLa cells. Infect Immun 62: 4900–4908
7. Clausen JD, Christiansen G, Holst HU, Birkelund S (1997) *Chlamydia trachomatis* utilizes the host cell microtubule network during early events of infection. Mol Microbiol 25: 441–449
8. Fan T, Lu H, Hu H, Shi L, McClarty GA, Nance DM, Greenberg AH, Zhong G (1998) Inhibition of apoptosis in chlamydia-infected cells: blockade of mitochondrial cytochrome C release and caspase activation. J Exp Med 187: 487–496
9. Fawaz FS, van Ooij C, Homola E, Mutka SC, Engel JN (1997) Infection with *Chlamydia trachomatis* alters the tyrosine phosphorylation and/or localization of several host cell proteins including cortacin. Infect Immun 65: 5301–5308
10. Herbold BC, Siston A, Bremer J, Kirkpatrik R, Wilbanks G, Fugedi P, Peto C, Cooper M (1997) Sulfated carbohydrate compounds prevent microbial adherence by sexually transmitted disease pathogens. Antimicrob Agents Chemother 41: 2776–2780
11. Knudsen K, Madsen AS, Mygind P, Christiansen G, Birkelund S (1999) Identification of two novel genes encoding 97- to 99- kilodalton outer membrane proteins of *Chlamydia pneumoniae*. Infect Immun 67: 375–383
12. Kuo CC, Takahashi N, Swanson AF, Ozeki Y, Hakomori SI (1996) An N-linked high mannose type oligosaccharide, expressed at the major outer membrane protein of *Chlamydia trachomatis*, mediates attachment and infectivity of the microorganism to HeLa cells. J Clin Invest 98: 2813–2818
13. Majeed M, Gustafsson M, Kihlstrom E, Stendahl O (1993) Roles of Ca2+ and actin in intracellular aggregation of *Chlamydia trachomatis* in eucaryotic cells. Infect Immun 61: 1406–1414
14. Rödel J, Groh A, Vogelsang H, Lehmann M, Hartmann M, Straube E (1998) IFN-β is produced by *Chlamydia trachomatis*-infected fibroblast-like synoviocytes and inhibits IFN-γ-induced HLA-DR expression. Infect Immun 66: 4491–4495
15. Rödel J, Straube E, Lungershausen W, Hartmann M, Groh A (1998) Secretion of cytokines by human synoviocytes during *in vitro* infection with *Chlamydia trachomatis*. J Rheumatol 11: 2161–2168

16. Rödel J, Groh A, Hartmann M, Schmidt KH, Lehmann M, Lungershausen W, Straube E (1999) Expression of interferon regulatory factors and indoleamine 3,3-dioxygenase in *Chlamydia trachomatis*-infected synovial fibroblasts. Med Microbiol Immunol 187: 205–212
17. Zaretzky FR, Pearce-Pratt R, Phillips DM (1995) Sulfated polyanions block *Chlamydia trachomatis* infection of cervix-derived human epithelia. Infect Immun 63: 3520–3526

1.2
Biology, immunology and persistence of *Chlamydia pneumoniae*: Links to chronic disease

G.I. Byrne and M.V. Kalayoglu

Chlamydiae are not typical prokaryotic organisms. They exhibit unique attributes not seen in other bacteria but relate directly to the sorts of diseases these organisms cause and their specific mode of pathogenesis. For example, *chlamydiae* not only are restricted to an obligate intracellular existence within the confines of a membrane-bound vesicle (inclusion) in the cytoplasm of susceptible host cells, but also they undergo morphologic, biochemical and physiologic changes during the course of their intracellular existence that impact directly the degree of host tissue damage at the site of infection. Their intracellular development can lead to either a productive infection or generation of a more chronic, persistent state, depending on the specific micro-environmental conditions of the infected host cell. Productive chlamydial growth involves host cell invasion by the environmentally stable elementary body (EB) followed by differentiation to the metabolically active reticulate body (RB). Growth and replication of RB then proceeds by binary fission. The cycle is completed when the greatly expanded number of RB differentiate back to EB and are released to infect new susceptible host cells. However, other growth options also exist for *chlamydiae* that extend the definition of intracellular chlamydial development to choices beyond orderly transitions between EB and RB. Study of cell culture systems [1–4] and observations *in vivo* [5–8] demonstrate that chlamydial growth may manifest in a whole spectrum of novel ways. For example, Moulder et al. [9] identified a cryptic form of chlamydial existence that may serve to perpetuate these organisms intracellularly in an unrecognizable form for extended periods of time. Similarly, intracellular RB may be induced to enter a non-replicative, noninfectious stage that results in a persistent, long-term relationship with the infected host cell and that partially duplicates events associated with chronic chlamydial infections. This non-productive growth stage has been termed persistence [1] and is characterized as a form of stressed chlamydial growth since stress response proteins such as Hsp60 are produced in elevated amounts as compared with the production of structural proteins under similar growth conditions. The full range of stimuli that can cause *chlamydiae* to enter the persistent state are not definitively known, but host cell activation by immune regulated cytokines, growth at elevated (39–42°C) temperatures and nutrient depletion appear to be three stress-related conditions that trigger persistence. It is noteworthy that persistence is not an irreversible process since removal of inducing stimuli results in resumption of the productive chlamydial growth cycle. *In vivo* evidence for chlamydial persistence also has recently emerged. Numerous clinical observations have been made to support the hypothesis that chlamydial persistence contributes to the chronic disease state. Relevant observations have been made from clinical conditions as diverse as arthritis [5], upper genital tract infections [6], trachoma [7], Alzheimer's disease [8] and atherosclerosis [10]. An important correlate of persistence and the disease process caused by *chlamydiae* involves the production of stress response proteins during persistent growth. Chlamydial stress response proteins have been associated with the pathologic consequences of chronic chlamydial diseases and will provide the focal point for data and experimental systems summarized here as these studies apply to the pathogenesis of atherosclerosis in the context of *C. pneumoniae* infection.

Chronic chlamydial diseases: *C. pneumoniae* and atherosclerosis

The spectrum of important and significant human chlamydial infectious diseases continues to expand. It is not only clear that *C. trachomatis* continues to be the most commonly encountered sexually transmitted bacterial infection (4 million new cases each year in the USA) but also the young women (15–19 year old adolescents) who have the highest rates of infection regardless of demographics or location are most likely to develop pelvic inflammatory disease (PID) and infertility during child bearing years [11]. In addition, the more recently described human respiratory pathogen, *C. pneumoniae*, has been associated with the induction and development of cardiovascular disease in a variety of studies using a number of criteria [12–20]. A key factor that serves to link upper genital tract disease sequelae in women and cardiovascular disease in both men and women is the well documented chronic nature of chlamydial infections that results when infections remain untreated or unrecognized [13–19]. Growth options available to *chlamydiae* in addition to the orderly alternation of elementary bodies (EB) and reticulate bodies (RB) have been described under numerous cell culture systems over the years [21–38] and some of these more esoteric states of intracellular chlamydial development have been suggested to contribute to chronic infections. We have made some contributions to this area of investigation by suggesting that immune response-regulated cytokines can cause at least some strains of *C. trachomatis* to enter a nonproductive growth state characterized by its reversibility, its long-term duration and its tendency to result in production of elevated stress response protein (Hsp60) amounts. It is significant that chlamydial Hsp60 has previously been implicated as a mediator of ocular and genital chronic disease pathology by virtue of its antigenicity [39–49] and more recently as a direct activator of mononuclear inflammatory cells in cardiovascular disease [50, 51].

Young and Elliot [52] have provided a useful overview that describes how stress proteins can be involved in infectious disease pathology based on observations showing that these proteins are up-regulated by both pathogens and the host under conditions of stress and Hsp's are major immunologic targets due to their intrinsic antigenicity and abundance. The possibility also exists for cross-reactive immune responses due to the high level of Hsp conservation between various pathogens. Thus, for infectious diseases involving exaggerated immune stimulation, Hsp reactivity can be a significant contributor. In addition, since eukaryotic stress proteins share a large degree of amino acid similarity with their microbial counterparts, autoimmunity may play a role in stress protein-related aspects of infectious disease pathogenesis.

It is significant that stress response proteins may exhibit disease-provoking mechanisms that extend beyond their well-documented role as antigens. Retzlaff et al. [53] reported that Hsp60 from *Legionella pneumophila* directly induced IL-1 mRNA via protein kinase C signaling. This observation is interesting in that it provides evidence that host cells are equipped with Hsp60 recognizing receptors to initiate signal transduction systems. Surface receptors to Hsp60 were further substantiated by Garduno et al. [54]) who showed that Hsp60 is surface-exposed on *L. pneumophila* and mediates invasion into HeLa cells via specific receptor-ligand interactions. The observations by Kol et al. [50, 51] showing that chlamydial Hsp60 directly stimulates induction of macrophage matrix metalloproteinase and vascular cell adhesion molecules suggests a direct signaling role for chlamydial Hsp60.

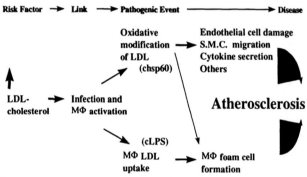

Figure 1: *Chlamydia pneumoniae* and atherosclerosis. Links between a known risk factor (elevated LDL, two possible chlamydial virulence factors (LPS and Hsp60) and the disease process (foam cell formation and oxidative-mediated tissue damage)

Chlamydial Hsp60 and the chronic disease process

Kol et al. [50] provided key insight for the macrophage activating capacity of Hsp60 and its association with atherosclerosis. We have recently investigated the possibility that chlamydial Hsp60 might cause direct activation of human monocyte-derived macrophages in ways that also relate to atherogenesis. We directed our attention to measuring oxidative modification of low density lipoprotein (LDL), an event with known pathologic potential in atherosclerotic lesions involving a well defined risk factor for cardiovascular disease with an infectious agent (*chlamydiae*). The experimental scheme and summary of the results are presented in figure form above (Figure 1). The data show that chlamydial Hsp60 (but not Hsp10 – data not shown) can cause macrophages to oxidatively modify LDL via a mechanism independent of respiratory burst activity. Interestingly, it appears that chlamydial Hsp60 and chlamydial LPS both are involved in different aspects of macrophage modulation related to atheroma development. A key area for investigation now will be to establish if Hsp60 can directly induce changes in macrophages and other cell types that may be important to the development of chronic sequelae of chlamydial infection.

A remarkable aspect of the emerging details concerning how Hsp60 may contribute to the disease process is that if Hsp60 is actually functioning as a direct signal transducer (immune modulator) in macrophages and possibly other cell types, then this suggests that an Hsp60-specific receptor must be present on affected cells.

Summary

The intent of this overview was to suggest some of the ways in which *C. pneumoniae* and chlamydial heat shock proteins may contribute to the development and progression of atherosclerosis. Data are emerging to suggest that chlamydial stress response proteins play a role in the induction and development of inflammatory events associated with atheromatous changes, at least as defined in cell culture systems. It is also significant, however, to note that chlamydial Hsp60 has actually been identified as being associated with human atherosclerotic tissue [50].

The continuous presence of chlamydial stress response proteins during chronic infection or as a result of repeated infections over time can influence the disease process in at least three ways. First, these proteins are antigenic. The immune responses elicited may directly result in tissue damage at the site of infection or may cause induction of cross reactive immune responses involving host heat shock protein homologues and thus the induction of autoimmunity. These two possibilities should be further distinguishable by continued careful analysis of T and B cell epitopes involved in eliciting cell mediated responses and antibody production. The third way in which chlamydial stress response proteins may participate in the disease process is by direct activation of mononuclear phagocytes and other responsive cells. This interesting possibility involving these proteins acting as direct immunomodulators, in a manner very similar to the well-known bacterial immunomodulator, LPS, may eventually have much more broadly applicable significance than has been described here. Additional disease promoting activities of chlamydial stress response proteins will no doubt emerge from the study of infectious causes of atherosclerosis and as details are discovered concerning how these microbial virulence factors function in ways that promote disease.

References

1. Beatty WL, Morrison RP, Byrne GI (1994) Persistent chlamydiae: from cell culture to a paradigm for chlamydial pathogenesis. Microbiol Rev 58: 686–699
2. Coles AM, Reynolds DJ, Harper A, Devitt A, Pearce JH (1993) Low-nutrient induction of abnormal chlamydial development: a novel component of chlamydial pathogenesis? FEMS Microbiol Lett 106: 193–200

3. Johnson FWA, Hobson D (1977) The effect of penicillin on genital strains of *Chlamydia trachomatis* in tissue culture. J Antimicrob Chemother 3: 49–56
4. Hatch TP (1975) Competition between Chlamydia psittaci and L cells for host isoleucine pools: a limiting factor in chlamydial multiplication. Infect Immun 12: 211–220
5. Beutler AM, Whittum-Hudson JA, Nanagara R, Schumacher HR, Hudson AP (1994) Intracellular location of inapparently infecting Chlamydia in synovial tissue from patients with Reiter's syndrome. Immunol Res 13: 163–171
6. Campbell LA, Patton DL, Moore DE, Cappuccio AL, Mueller BA, Wang SP (1993) Detection of *Chlamydia trachomatis* deoxyribonucleic acid in women with tubal infertility. Fertil Steril 59: 45–50
7. Ward M, Bailey R, Lesley A, Kajbaf M, Robertson J, Mabey D (1990) Persisting inapparent chlamydial infection in a trachoma endemic community in The Gambia. Scand J Infect Dis Suppl 69: 137–148
8. Balin BJ, Gerard HC, Arking EJ, Appelt DM, Branigan PJ, Abrams JT, Whittum-Hudson J, Hudson AP (1998) Identification and localization of *Chlamydia pneumoniae* in the Alzheimer's brain. Med Microbiol Immunol 187: 23–42
9. Moulder JW, Levy NJ, Schulman RP (1980) Persistent infection of mouse fibroblasts (L cells) with Chlamydia psittaci: evidence for a cryptic chlamydial form. Infect Immun 30: 874–883
10. Kol A, Sukhova GK, Lichtman AH, Libby P (1998) Chlamydial heat shock protein 60 localizes in human atheroma and regulates macrophage tumor necrosis factor-α and matrix metalloproteinase expression. Circulation 98: 300–307
11. Anonymous (1998) Chlamydial infection. NIAID Fact Sheet. NIH Office of Communications and Public Liaison. Bethesda, MD pp 1-3
12. Gupta S, Leatham E, Carrington D, Mendall M, Kaski J, Camm J (1997) Elevated *Chlamydia pneumoniae* antibodies, cardiovascular events, and azithromycin in male survivors of myocardial infarction. Circulation 96: 404–407
13. Gurfinkel E, Bozovich G, Daroca A, Beck E, Mautner B (1997) Randomized trial of roxithromycin in non-Q-wave coronary syndromes-Roxis pilot study. Lancet 350: 404–407
14. Jackson L, Campbell L, Kuo C, Rodriguez D, Lee A, Grayston J (1997) Isolation of *Chlamydia pneumoniae* from a carotid endarterectomy specimen. J Infect Dis 176: 292–295
15. Kuo C, Gown A, Benditt E, Grayston J (1993) Detection of *Chlamydia pneumoniae* in aortic lesions of atherosclerosis by immunocytochemical stain. Arterioscler Thromb 13: 1501–1504
16. Kuo C, Grayston J, Campbell LA, Goo Y, Wissler W, Benditt E (1995) *Chlamydia pneumoniae* (TWAR) in coronary arteries of young adults. Proc Natl Acad Sci USA 92: 6911–6914
17. Moazed T, Kuo C, Grayston T, Campbell L (1997) Murine models of *Chlamydia pneumoniae* infection and atherosclerosis. J Infect Dis 175: 883–890
18. Muhlestein J, Anderson J, Hammond E, Zhao L, Trehan S, Schwobe E, Carlquist J (1998) Infection with *Chlamydia pneumoniae* accelerates the development of atherosclerosis and treatment with azithromycin prevents it in a rabbit model. Circulation 97: 633–636
19. Saikku P, Leinonen M, Tenkanen L, Linnanmaki E, Ekman M, Manninen V, Manttari M, Frick M, Huttunen M (1992) Chronic *Chlamydia pneumoniae* infection as a risk factor for coronary heart disease in the Helsinki Heart Study. Ann Intern Med 116: 273–278

20. Shor A, Kuo C, Patton D (1992) Detection of *Chlamydia pneumoniae* in coronary arterial fatty streaks and atheromatous plaques. S Afr Med J 82: 158–161
21. Allen I, Hatch T, Pearce J (1985) Influence of cysteine deprivation on chlamydial differentiation from reproductive to infective life-cycle forms. J Gen Microbiol 131: 3171–3177
22. Allen I, Pearce J (1983) Amino acid requirements *Chlamydia trachomatis* and *C. psittaci* strains in McCoy cells: relationship with clinical syndrome and host origin. J Gen Microbiol 129: 2001–2007
23. Armstrong J, Reed S (1967) Fine structure of lymphogranuloma venereum agent and the effects of penicillin and 5-fluorouracil. J Gen Microbiol 46: 435–444
24. Bader J, Morgan H (1958) Latent viral infection of cells in tissue culture. VI. Role of amino acids, glutamine and glucose in psittacosis virus propagation in L cells. J Exp Med 106: 617–629
25. Bader J, Morgan H (1961) Latent viral infection of cells in tissue culture. VII. Role of water soluble vitamins in psittacosis virus propagation in L cells. J Exp Med 113: 271–281
26. Coles A, Reynolds DJ, Harper A, Devitt A, Pearce J (1993) Low-nutrient induction of abnormal chlamydial development: a novel component of chlamydial pathogenesis? FEMS Lett 106: 193–200
27. Galasso G, Manire G (1961) Effect of antiserum and antibiotics on persistent infection of HeLa cells with meningopneumonitis virus. J Immunol 86: 382–385
28. Hatch T (1975) Competition between *Chlamydia psittaci* and L cells for host isoleucine pools: a limiting factor in chlamydial multiplication. Infect Immun 12: 211–220
29. Hatch T, Allen I, Pearce J (1984) Structural and polypeptide differences between envelopes of infective and reproductive life cycle forms of Chlamydia spp. J Bacteriol 157: 13–20
30. Holland S, Hudson A, Bobo L, Whittum-Hudson J, Viscidi R, Quinn T, Taylor H (1992) Demonstration of chlamydial RNA and DNA during a culture negative state. Infect Immun 60: 2040–2047
31. Matsumoto A, Manire G (1970) Electron microscopic observations on the effects of penicillin on the morphology of *Chlamydia psittaci*. J Bacteriol 101: 278–285
32. Morgan H (1956) Latent viral infection of cells in tissue culture. I. Studies on latent infection of chick embryo tissues with psittacosis virus. J Exp Med 103: 37–47
33. Moulder J, Levy N, Schulman R (1980) Persistent infection of mouse fibroblasts (L cells) with *Chlamydia psittaci*: evidence for a cryptic chlamydial form. Infect Immun 30: 874–883
34. Perez-Martinez J, Storz J (1985) Persistent infection of L cells with an ovine abortion strain of *Chlamydia psittaci*. Infect Immun 50: 453–458
35. Pollard M, Sharon N (1963) Induction of prolonged latency in psittacosis infected cells by aminopterin. Proc Soc Exp Biol Med 112: 51–55
36. Sarov I, Geron E, Shemer-Avni Y, Manor E, Zvillich M, Wallach D, Schmidtz E, Holtman H (1991) Implications for persistent chlamydial infections of phagocyte-microorganism interplay. Eur J Clin Microbiol Infect Dis 10: 119–123
37. Tanimi Y, Yamada Y (1973) Miniature cell formation in *Chlamydia psittaci*. J Bacteriol 114: 408–412
38. Ward M, Salari H (1982) Control mechanisms governing the infectivity of *Chlamydia trachomatis* for HeLa cells: modulation by cyclic nucleotides prostaglandins and calcium. J Gen Micro 128: 639–650
39. Brunham R, Peeling R (1994) *Chlamydia trachomatis* antigens: role in immunity and pathogenesis. Infect Agents Dis 3: 218–233

40. Sziller I, Witkin S, Ziegert M, Csapo Z, Ujhazy A, Papp Z (1998) Serologic responses of patients with ectopic pregnancy to epitopes of the *Chlamydia trachomatis* 60 kDa heat shock protein. Human Reprod 13: 1088–1093
41. Domeika M, Domeika K, Paavonen J, Mardh P, Witkin S (1998) Humoral immune response to conserved epitopes of *Chlamydia trachomatis* and human 60-kDa heat-shock protein in women with pelvic inflammatory disease. J Infect Dis 177: 714–719
42. Eckert L, Hawes S, Wolner-Hanssen P, Money D, Peeling R, Brunham R, Stevens V, Eschenbach D, Stamm W (1997) Prevalence and correlates of antibody to chlamydial heat shock protein in women attending sexually transmitted disease clinics and women with confirmed pelvic inflammatory disease. J Infect Dis 175: 1453–1458
43. Money D, Hawes S, Eschenbach D, Peeling R, Brunham R, Wolner-Hanssen P, Stamm W (1997) Antibodies to the chlamydial 60 kd heat-shock protein are associated with laparoscopically confirmed perihepatitis. Am J Obstet Gynecol 176: 870–877
44. Toye B, Laferriere C, Claman P, Jessamine P, Peeling R (1993) Association between antibody to the chlamydial heat-shock protein and tubal infertility. J Infect Dis 168: 1236–1240
45. Witkin S, Jeremias J, Toth M, Ledger W (1993) Cell-mediated immune response to the recombinant 57 kDa heat shock protein of *Chlamydia trachomatis* in women with salpingitis. J Infect Dis 167: 1379–1383
46. Morrison R, Lyng K, Caldwell H (1989) Chlamydial disease pathogenesis. Ocular hypersensitivity elicited by a genus-specific 57 kd protein. J Exp Med 169: 663–675
47. Patton D, Cosgrove-Sweeney Y, Kuo C (1994) Demonstration of delayed hypersensitivity in *Chlamydia trachomatis* salpingitis in monkeys: a pathogenic mechanism of tubal damage. J Infect Dis 169: 680–683
48. Taylor H, Johnson S, Schachter J, Caldwell H, Prendergast R (1987) Pathogenesis of trachoma: the stimulus for inflammation. J Immunol 138: 3023–3027
49. Witkin S, Jeremias J, Toth M, Ledger W (1994) Proliferative response to conserved epitopes of the *Chlamydia trachomatis* and human 60-kilodalton heat-shock proteins by lymphocytes from women with salpingitis. Am J Obstet Gynecol 171: 445–460
50. Kol A, Sukhova G, Lichtman A, Libby P (1998) Chlamydial heat shock protein 60 localizes in human atheroma and regulates macrophage tumor-necrosis factor and matrix metalloproteinase expression. Circulation 98: 300–307
51. Kol A, Bourcier V, Lichtman AH, Libby P (1999) Chlamydial and human heat shock protein 60s activate human vascular endothelium, smooth muscle cells, and macrophages. J Clin Invest 103: 571–577
52. Young R, Elliot V (1989) Stress proteins, infection, and immune surveillance. Cell 59: 5–8
53. Retzlaff C, Yamamoto V, Okubo S, Hoffman P, Friedman H, Klein T (1996) *Legionella pneumophila* heat-shock protein-induced increase of interleukin 1 mRNA involves protein kinase C signalling in macrophages. Immunology 89: 281–288
54. Garduno R, Faulkner V, Trevors M, Vats N, Hoffman P (1998) Immunolocalization of Hsp60 in *Legionella pneumophila*. J Bacteriol 180: 505–513

Discussion

Maass:

You have shown you can recover Chlamydia by culture from a persistent state. Is it also possible to recover them from the persistent state in macrophages? We have tried this and see aberrant inclusions in the macrophages for about 30 days but we can't recover them and in fact we can't eliminate them with antibiotics.

Byrne:

You are referring specifically to *C. pneumoniae* in macrophages? We haven't looked to that. That is interesting that they are non-recoverable from macrophages. What we are doing actually is adding the infected macrophages to a human diploid adult endothelium monolayer. We are wondering whether or not you can transfer the infection to another cell type that might better support a productive infection. I think that again when you look at the dynamics of the situation that would be an area that could allow for a better chance to recover organisms.

Klos:

Is the foam cell formation which you observe dependent on Chlamydia LPS or is it a more general phenomenon which you could also achieve if other bacteria only would persist in atherosclerotic plaques?

Byrne:

Yes, it is general. LPS works in this assay. There are some features that I am sure Dr. Brade can expand upon that make chlamydial LPS very unique. It is kind of a wimpy LPS in a lot of ways. Chlamydial LPS is not going to induce endotoxemia if you use it *in vivo*. It certainly is not a good inducer of TNF-alpha in the presence of LPS-binding protein (serum). You have to put this in the context of where the events we are studying are actually happening in the body during an infection. We are talking here about LPS which is normally thought of as a very acute mediator, functioning in a very chronic state. But since chlamydial LPS is wimpy and doesn't do a lot of activation, it is still able to induce foam cells, whereas if you had some other gram-negatives present under similar circumstances, there would be more acute events going on much more rapidly.

The second thing is that Chlamydia is at the scene of the crime. There are only two organisms as far as I know that have been consistently associated with the atherosclerotic lesion. One is cytomegalovirus and the other is *Chlamydia pneumoniae*. So you have an organism that is present and armed in ways that are generic (Hsp60 and LPS). But still it is there and capable of doing the changes that are associated with atherogenesis. Whether there are other organisms that are going to emerge that can do the same changes or whether this is kind of what Dr. Libby refers as the 'echo effect' where you have some infectious process going on at a distant site and it echoes back to the atheromatous tissue, I don't know. These are things we need to study *in vivo* using animal models which we will hear about later today, to extend the argument to a more realistic situation.

Brade:

Perhaps I should have saved my comment for tomorrow but it may be relevant for some other talks. First I wanted to ask: the experiments which you have done with the isolated chlamydial LPS, is that the LPS from Doug Golenbock that was isolated from *Chlamydia trachomatis* serotype F?

Byrne:
Yes.

Brade:
It is definitely known, although not everyone is aware of it, that LPS and LPS in Chlamydia are not the same. We are usually looking to it as an antigen, and we have learned that there is an epitope which is shared by the whole genome for all of the four species. But concerning the lipid portion of the LPS and even in the KDO regions there are differences. *Psittaci* is different from *trachomatis*.

Byrne:
Do you know about *C. pneumoniae*?

Brade:
We do not know about *C. pneumoniae* but there is very good evidence that in *C. pneumoniae* there is something which is not present in other lipopolysaccharides. Remember the paper we published with Elena Peterson on a monoclonal antibody which is able to bind in *in vitro* assays on a genus-specific level but which at the same time is able to neutralize *C. pneumoniae* on a species-specific and even on a strain-specific level. We do not know the structural elements responsible for this reaction pattern, but we should just keep in mind, LPS within this species is not the same.

Then we come to the more general point: From the enterobacterial work on endotoxins we have learned that a single fatty acid can determine whether a lipid A is an agonist or an antagonist in terms of inducing proinflammatory cytokines. In *E. coli* a hexa-acyl species is a strong agonist for human monocytes, whereas a tetra-acyl specimen is a strong antagonist. With Chlamydia we know from the work of Kaski that was published last year that the distribution of fatty acids focuses on two main molecular species with four and five fatty acids, and these two molecules are present as a mixture. From data that we have generated in tissue-culture grown Chlamydia we know that the ratio of these two fractions varies very much. If you envisage that one of these molecules is an agonist and the other is an antagonist and that the ratio of these two species depends on the environmental conditions where these Chlamydia multiply, I think you can imagine everything in this picture. So we should just be open to know that, independent of the report that chlamydial LPS is not a good inducer of proinflammatory cytokines, under these conditions of the inflammation in the cell wall it can behave differently and be a very strong agonist.

Byrne:
Right. I appreciate those points. I knew I was in trouble when I started talking about LPS and Dr. Brade was in the front row. At this point we knew that heat-killed Chlamydia caused induction of foam cells. We couldn't get *C. pneumoniae* LPS but wanted to begin the experimental process in a way that made sense to us. So we had to use *C. trachomatis* LPS and we were lucky to get it. But in fact *C. pneumoniae* does it in a way that is heat stable. I think we are on the right track,

but if we ever get enough of the right LPS molecules to study agonist/antagonist effects and how the details of LPS structure relate to activities we are seeing, then I expect these studies with synthetic chlamydial LPS to provide a wealth of interesting data. This is going to have to wait until we have the molecules, and I hear that there may be some lipid A on the horizon.

Stille:

Did you look at calcium metabolism of cells? In clinical atherosclerosis calcification plays a far greater role than real lipoidosis, and so-called atheroma do not contain great amounts of lipids, maybe up only to 5 %. But old atherosclerotic tissue may have up to 50 % calcium and there can be gross calcification. I would like to remind you of the trivial German name for calcification of arteries: "*Arterienverkalkung*" is an historical name.

Byrne:

I would, however, strongly disagree with the point that lipid accumulation plays only a minor role in atheroma development.

Stille:

But it has to be expected that something is going on on a cellular basis concerning calcium channels or whatever.

Byrne:

That is again an interesting point. It wasn't our point though but another set of studies that could be done. Certainly you wouldn't argue about fatty streaks and early changes relating to the presence of foam cells, the presence of lipids in the developing lesion. We are talking about very early events. We can argue about whether Chlamydia plays a role early, late, never, whatever. But we are talking about early events right now. I think your question relates to other interesting activities that need to be looked at. But that is not where we are at the moment.

Klos:

It didn't become clear to me from your slides: In which of the different cells which are important in the context of atherosclerosis do you actually observe long-term persistence?

Byrne:

We haven't studied a long-term persistence with *C. pneumoniae* the way we have with *C. trachomatis*. We have restricted our analysis right now to macrophages. They do go persistent in macrophages. Important questions are how long they remain persistent and what other cell types may be involved. We have at least one other cell type in mind to evaluate, the endothelial cell.

Straube:

Is the foam cell formation dependent on the intracellular Chlamydia or is this dependent on an external LPS because chlamydia-infected macrophages express CD14 in a higher amount?

Byrne:

The Chlamydia do get taken up when we see foam cell formation happen. But you don't have to have that. LPS will work just like *C. pneumoniae* will. But when you are using *C. pneumoniae*, they do get taken up. We have not directly analyzed for modulation of CD14.

Hammerschlag:

Actually in the issue of chronic infection we have been able in Hep2 cells to have two strains, TW183 and CM1, which have been going on for about one to two years in tissue where you see your cycles of lysis and regrowth of the cells. Every couple of days we just put the cells on new medium, we don't add new cells, we don't add new Chlamydia and it keeps going. What you see on the supernatant in these cells opposed to acutely infected is a very increased expression of a number of cytokines, and with antibiotics using even ofloxacin four times the amount for MIC, you get reduction in the IFU but never elimination, still sort of baseline 10 to the three IFU per ml. For Chlamydia we don't know what's happening to the *in vitro* susceptibilities at that point. We are looking at it because after azithromycin treatment in patients with pneumonia we had a few strains with the MICs looking like they were beginning to creep up. At least there were two-fold increases which is something that we generally see, and four-fold increases to dilutions which we had not really seen before. We have seen those that had been stable. We are continuing to kind of play with this, but can we adapt the more recent isolates by the other cell lines? It just goes on and on.

Byrne:

This raises another point, too. I have referred to one additional growth option that Chlamydia has: the persisting form. But there are many others. In the 1970s Jim Moulder described cryptic Chlamydia: cells were infected but there was no evidence for this at all other than the fact that every month or so Chlamydia would bloom out of them and they were resistant to superinfection, so you couldn't infect them with fresh Chlamydia. These other possible growth options just haven't been elaborated in experimental systems very well. We tend to think that Chlamydia has an orderly process for growing intracellularly, but I don't think it really is that orderly most of the time *in vivo*. There are many different ways. The Chlamydia can hang around for long periods of time.

The second point is about antibiotics and resistance. We are not talking about acquiring resistance in Chlamydia, rather we are talking about a growth state that makes them less susceptible to eradication. The Chlamydia that grow out of the azithromycin-treated cultures are just as susceptible to azithromycin as when they are growing normally. They are not getting resistant to azithromycin. They are just less likely to be eradicated when they are in the persistent state.

1.3
Animal models for *Chlamydia pneumoniae* infection

M. Leinonen and P. Saikku

Chlamydia pneumoniae is transmitted from man to man and no animal species has been implicated in its circulation [1]. However, chlamydial strains closely related to *C. pneumoniae* have been found in animals [2, 3], and the disease can be easily transmitted into experimental animals. Thus far, three animal models for *C. pneumoniae* infection have been evaluated. *C. pneumoniae* is capable to infect mice, monkeys and rabbits by different challenge routes, e.g., by intranasal, intravenous and subcutaneous inoculations.

Monkey models for *C. pneumoniae* infection

Different monkey species, baboons as well as rhesus and cynomolgus monkeys, have been infected by using different challenge routes with *C. pneumoniae*, strain TWAR [4, 5]. The infected animals do not develop any clinical disease, both organisms can be recovered from the nasopharynx after inoculation. The infection persisted for a prolonged period and, interestingly, in cynomolgus monkeys the intranasally inoculated agent was demonstrated also in rectal swabs, pointing to a systemic spread [5].

Mouse models for *C. pneumoniae* infection

Mouse models to study immunopathogenesis and defense mechanism in *C. pneumoniae* infection have been developed [6, 7, 8, 9, 10]. There are differences both in the susceptibility of different mouse strains to *C. pneumoniae* infection and in the virulence of different *C. pneumoniae* strains. We have shown in our studies that NIH mice are most homogeneously infected with *C. pneumoniae* after intranasal inoculation with a relatively small challenge dose (10^5 inclusion forming units). Furthermore, in our mouse model *C. pneumoniae*, Kajaani 6, epidemic Finnish strain, has been shown to be more virulent than the original TW183 strain or interepidemic Finnish strain, Helsinki 12 [7].

Mice develop a strong antibody response against *C. pneumoniae* peaking at 3 to 4 weeks after intranasal challenge [7]. *C. pneumoniae* can be isolated from lung tissues for more than two weeks after the challenge and there is an inverse relationship between isolation yield and specific antibody level. In the model of Yang et al. [8] primary infection induced an acute, patchy pneumonia with polymorphonuclear leukocytes and exudate in lung alveoli and bronchi that in two weeks turned to a predominantly monocytic infiltration. In our model [6], using ten times lower inoculum of the bacteria – which probably is a clinically more relevant dose – no purulent pneumonia was seen. Histology showed bronchopneumonia that was characterized by a chronic type of inflammation with perivascular and peribronchial lymphocyte infiltrations and minor interstitial inflammation. The changes developed more slowly than in Yang's model, but were as long-lasting and stayed demonstrable for several weeks after the challenge. Our more recent data [9] on the reinfections in the mice indicate that chlamydial cultures are positive only for a couple of days after the rechallenge. However, the inflammatory changes in the lungs are as strong and long-lasting and develop earlier than the changes seen in primary infection. Further, *C. pneumoniae* DNA can be demonstrated in lungs by PCR and *in situ* DNA hybridization after the cultures have turned negative. When convalescent or hyperimmune serum is given intraperitoneally prior to the intranasal challenge, Chlamydia cultures stay negative, but the lung histology shows acute pneumonia with polymorphonuclear leukocytes [9]. After *C. pneumoniae* infection, Chlamydia may remain in the body in a latent state during which it can be reactivated by immunosuppression. By using the study protocol described by Yang et al. [11] for *C. trachomatis*, it has been shown that when mice were treated with cortisone after recovery from primary infection, i.e. at the time when no Chlamydia could be found any more by culture, *C. pneumoniae* could be reisolated from lung tissue two weeks after the cortisone treatment was started [12, 13].

C. pneumoniae has been shown to spread systemically in mice after intranasal inoculation. *C. pneumoniae* can be isolated from spleen and peritoneal macrophages as frequently as from the lungs of intranasally infected mice [14]. Our preliminary studies have also shown that *C. pneumoniae* can be demonstrated by PCR from the heart tissue of NIH mice even over 1 month after the primary intranasal challenge.

Rabbit model for *C. pneumoniae* infection

New Zealand White (NZW) rabbits, after intranasal or intratracheal inoculation of *C. pneumoniae*, develop respiratory disease with moderate interstitial pneumonia, bronchiolitis and vasculitis [15]. In repeatedly reinfected rabbits pulmonary microgranulomas, consisting of a central macrophage core surrounded by activated lymphocytes, are formed. Furthermore, also in the rabbit model, *C. pneumoniae* is able to spread systematically as indicated by demonstration of *C. pneumoniae* DNA by polymerase chain reaction in spleen tissue and peripheral blood mononuclear cells.

Animal models for *C. pneumoniae*-associated atherosclerosis

The Seattle group has published their results of mouse models for atherosclerosis [16]. They have used apolipoprotein (Apo)-E-deficient mice, which spontaneously develop atherosclerosis and C57BL/6J mice, which only develop atherosclerosis on atherogenic diet. Following single or multiple intranasal inoculations in Apo-E-deficient mice, *C. pneumoniae* was detected in lung, aorta and spleen for 20 weeks after inoculation in 25–100 % of mice. In the aorta *C. pneumoniae* were detected within the atherosclerotic lesions. In C57BL/6J *C. pneumoniae* was detected in the aorta only for 2 weeks in 8 % of mice. This suggested at least a tropism of *C. pneumoniae* to atheromatous lesions. Hu and his coworkers published their mouse model recently [17]. They used B6,129 mice with low density lipoprotein receptor deficiency, which with a high cholesterol diet spontaneously develop atherosclerosis. Mice were infected intranasally with *C. pneumoniae* AR39 strain or *C. trachomatis* Mouse Pneumonitis (MoPn) strain once a month for 9 months. The combination of high cholesterol diet and *C. pneumoniae* infection significantly increased the lesion areas and the lesion severity compared to high cholesterol diet only. Although both *C. pneumoniae* and MoPn antigens were present in aorta samples, *C. trachomatis* MoPn had no atherogenic effect.

It was also reported recently that *Chlamydia* infections and heart disease are linked by antigenic mimicry [18]. A peptide from the murine heart muscle α-myosin heavy chain which has sequence homology with chlamydial 60 kD cysteine-rich outer membrane protein was shown to induce autoimmune heart disease in mice, and injection of homologous chlamydial peptides also induced perivascular inflammation, fibrotic changes and blood vessel occlusion in the heart. This mechanism, however, may play a more important role in myocarditis and cardiomyopathy than in atherosclerosis.

The rabbit model seems to be very promising, too. Fong et al. [19] have showed that NZW rabbits infected with *C. pneumoniae*, besides developing pneumonia, also presented fatty streaks and grade III atherosclerotic lesions in aortas in 2 of 6 animals 1 to 2 weeks after infection. We have also infected NZW rabbits, fed with normal diet, intranasally with *C. pneumoniae* [20]. Reinfection was given three weeks later. Six of nine reinfected animals showed inflammatory changes consisting of intimal thickening or fibroid plaques resembling atherosclerosis within 2 to 4 weeks after reinfection. One rabbit even had calcified lesions. Immunohistochemistry for *C. pneumoniae* was positive in all these animals. The results suggest that *C. pneumoniae* infection is capable of inducing inflammatory atherosclerosis-like changes in the aorta of infected rabbits. Thus in both rabbit models, atherosclerotic changes developed after *C. pneumoniae* challenge, suggesting that *C. pneumoniae* infection of the arterial wall may initiate development of atherosclerosis. Muhlestein *et al.* [21] have also been successful with this animal model. They used three intranasal inoculations with *C. pneumoniae* and rabbits were fed with chow enriched with 0.25 % cholesterol, and they could show that *C. pneumoniae* accelerates intimal thickening and that weekly treatment with azithromycin after exposure prevents this acceleration.

Conclusions

Animal models seem to be of great importance in studying the pathogenesis of chronic infections caused by *C. pneumoniae*, not only in the respiratory but also in the cardiovascular system. They have already been used in therapeutic studies on acute infections [22, 23] and can in future be useful also in attempts to find a cure in chronic inflammations caused by this unique pathogen.

References

1. Kuo CC, Jackson LA, Campbell LA, Grayston JT (1995) *Chlamydia pneumoniae* (TWAR). Clin Microbiol Rev 8: 451–461
2. Girjes AA, Carrick FN, Lavin MF (1994) Remarkable sequence relatedness in the DNA encoding the major outer membrane protein of *Chlamydia psittaci* (koala type I) and *Chlamydia pneumoniae*. Gene 138: 139–142
3. Storey C, Lusher M, Yates P, Richmond S (1993) Evidence for *Chlamydia pneumoniae* of non-human origin. J Gen Microbiol 139: 2621–2626
4. Bell TA, Kuo CC, Wang SP, Grayston JT (1989) Experimental infection of baboons (Papio cynocephalus anubis) with *Chlamydia pneumoniae* strain TWAR. J Infect 19: 47–49
5. Holland SM, Taylor H, Gaydos CA, Kappus EW, Quinn TC (1990) Experimental infection with *Chlamydia pneumoniae* in nonhuman primates. Infect Immun 58: 593–597
6. Kishimoto T (1990) Studies on *Chlamydia pneumoniae*, strain TWAR infection. I. Experimental infection of *C. pneumoniae* in mice and serum antibodies against TWAR by MFA. J Jap Assoc Infect Dis 64: 124–131
7. Kaukoranta-Tolvanen SS, Laurila AL, Saikku P, Leinonen M, Liesirova L, Laitinen K (1993) Experimental infection of *Chlamydia pneumoniae* in mice. Microb Pathog 15: 293–302
8. Yang ZP, Kuo CC, Grayston JT (1993) A mouse model of *Chlamydia pneumoniae* strain TWAR pneumonitis. Infect Immun 61: 2037–2040
9. Kaukoranta-Tolvanen SS, Laurila A, Saikku P, Leinonen M, Laitinen K (1995) Experimental *Chlamydia pneumoniae* infection in mice: Effect of reinfection and passive immunization. Microb Pathog 18: 279–288
10. Yang ZP, Cummings PK, Patton DL, Kuo CC (1994) Ultrastructural lung pathology of experimental *Chlamydia pneumoniae* pneumonitis in mice. J Infect Dis 170: 464–467
11. Yang YS, Kuo CC, Chen WJ (1987) Reactivation of *Chlamydia trachomatis* lung infection in mice by cortisone. Infect Immun 39: 655–658
12. Malinverni R, Kuo CC, Campbell LA, Grayston JT (1995) Reactivation of *Chlamydia pneumoniae* lung infection in mice by cortisone. J Infect Dis 172: 593–594
13. Laitinen K, Laurila A, Leinonen M, Saikku P (1996) Reactivation of *Chlamydia pneumoniae* infection in mice by cortisone treatment. Infect Immun 64: 1488–1490
14. Yang ZP, Kuo CC, Grayston JT (1995) Systemic dissemination of *Chlamydia pneumoniae* following intranasal inoculation of mice. J Infect Dis 171: 736–738
15. Moazed TC, Kuo CC, Patton DL, Grayston JT, Campbell LA (1996) Experimental rabbit models of *Chlamydia pneumoniae* infection. Am J Pathol 148: 667–676
16. Moazed TC, Kuo CC, Grayston JT, Campbell LA (1997) Murine models of *Chlamydia pneumoniae* infection and atherosclerosis. J Infect Dis 175: 883–890
17. Hu H, Pierce GN, Zhong G (1999) The atherogenic effects of chlamydia are dependent on serum cholesterol and specific to *Chlamydia pneumoniae*. J Clin Invest 103: 747–753
18. Bachmaier K, Neu N, de la Maza LM, Pal S, Hassel A, Penninger JM (1999) Chlamydia infections and heart disease linked through antigenic mimicry. Science 283: 1335–1339
19. Fong IW, Chiu B, Viira E, Fong MW, Jang D, Mahony J (1997) Rabbit model for *Chlamydia pneumoniae* infection. J Clin Microbiol 35: 48–52
20. Laitinen K, Laurila A, Pyhälä L, Leinonen M, Saikku P (1997) *Chlamydia pneumoniae* infection induces inflammatory changes in the aortas of rabbits. Infect Immun 65: 4832–4835

21. Muhlestein JB, Anderson JL, Hammond EH, Zhao L, Trehan S, Schwobe BS, Carlquist JF (1998) Infection with *Chlamydia pneumoniae* accelerates the development of atherosclerosis and treatment with azithromycin prevents it in a rabbit model. Circulation 97: 633–636
22. Malinverni R, Kuo CC, Campbell LA, Lee A, Grayston JT (1995) Effects of two antibiotic regimens on course and persistence of experimental *Chlamydia pneumoniae* (TWAR) pneumonitis. Antimicrobial Agents Chemother 39: 45–49
23. Soejima R, Niki Y, Kishimoto T, Miyashita N, Kubota Y, Nakata K (1995) *In vitro* and *in vivo* activities of new fluoroquinolones against *Chlamydia pneumoniae*. Can J Infect Dis 6 (Suppl C): 354C

Discussion

Byrne:
Dr. Leinonen, getting back to your serology on the Hsp60 where you are looking at cross-reactivities as a potential mechanism. The other thing was that there wasn't much cross-reactivity to the human homology and I presume you use that because the mouse or rabbit wasn't available. I mean it didn't really cross-react with more of a species-specific homolog of Hsp60. I wonder if you could comment on that.

Leinonen:
We have measured antibodies also in humans. We have been using *C. pneumoniae*-specific Hsp60, mycobacterial Hsp65 and human Hsp60, and it is interesting that some patients have very high antibody levels against all these proteins. Then some people have antibodies mostly against mycobacterial Hsp and some have human Hsp60 antibodies. It is really very mixed up. I do not know which are the mechanisms playing a role there. We would like to look at antibody responses to specific peptides and cross-reactive peptides to see what is really happening.

Brade:
If you consider the data which Dr. Byrne showed us this morning, have you done or are you aware of others doing experiments in the CD40 knock-out mouse which is now available?

Leinonen:
Yes, we have been thinking that it would be a very interesting model but it has not been used yet.

Kurth:
There is now a relatively newly developed knock-out mouse, namely for TNF-α receptor, which is said to be without protection against all intracellularly growing bacteria. Has anyone used it for Chlamydia animal models? Or would you expect that these mice will die rapidly?

Leinonen:
Possibly so. We have not tested.

Essig:
Did you examine scid-mice which are lacking functional B and T-cells if they develop atherosclerosis?

Leinonen:
We have not tested and I do not know if anybody else has tried it. But we would like to have some kind of model for acute myocardial infarction, and we saw that in SLE-prone immune-complex mice (MRL-mice) LPS can induce acute myocardial infarctions. We infected these mice with *C. pneumoniae* and we found that they had huge infiltrations of all kinds of inflammatory cells in their lungs, and they died so rapidly that we could not see any acute myocardial infarctions in those mice.

Ossewaarde:
We have learned from Dr. Byrne that Hsp60 and Chlamydia LPS might play a very important role in atherogenesis in animal models. You showed recent studies in which *C. pneumoniae* and the mouse pneumonitis strain were used to infect animals, and *C. pneumoniae* enhances atherosclerosis but mouse pneumonitis does not. And mouse pneumonitis also has Hsp60 and Chlamydial LPS. Could someone comment on these results?

Leinonen:
As I said, *C. pneumoniae* may have some extra features which contribute to the pathogenesis. Furthermore, *C. pneumoniae* is sitting in the atherosclerotic lesions. For instance, *C. trachomatis* is usually causing a genital infection, and possibly the mouse pneumonitis strain is not spread systemically in the mice. I think that this is an important feature, as Dr. Byrne mentioned in his talk as well.

1.4
Molecular biology and serodiagnostics of *Chlamydia pneumoniae* – potential way to a vaccine

G. Christiansen, A.S. Madsen, T. Boesen, K. Hjernø, L. Daugaard,
K. Knudsen, P. Mygind, S. Birkelund

Introduction

In *Chlamydia*, the obligate intracellular human pathogen with a unique biphasic life cycle, surface structures are of importance for induction of uptake in host cells, for protection of *Chlamydiae* at the extracellular stage, and as immunogens to which the host's humoral immune response is directed. In contrast to *C. trachomatis*, in which a major immunogen is the surface-localized major outer membrane protein (MOMP) [1], this protein is non-immunogenic in *C. pneumoniae* infections [2]. *C. pneumoniae* causes upper respiratory tract infections [3], pneumonia, and is suspected to play a role in the development of atherosclerosis [4, 5]. Proteins that contain only conformational epitopes cover the surface of *C. pneumoniae* [6]. We have previously characterized a gene family of at least four members that encodes surface-localized proteins [7, 8]. We obtained the clones by screening an expression library with an antibody (pAbdOmc) generated against purified, SDS-denatured *C. pneumoniae* outer membrane complex (Omc) proteins [9], hereby obtaining antibodies to linear epitopes that in native Omc were non-immunogenic [7]. By using antibodies generated to both linear and conformational epitopes of various parts of the recombinant proteins, we showed (i) that the proteins were the 97–99 kDa Omc proteins not present in *C. trachomatis* Omc [6]; (ii) that the 97–99 kDa proteins migrated as 73 kDa in unheated samples for SDS-PAGE; (iii) that these proteins were the major immunogens in experimentally infected mice; and (iv) that the proteins were present on the surface of *C. pneumoniae* [7].

The GGAI gene family

By comparison of the *C. pneumoniae* genome sequenced by R. Stephens [10] to be found at http://chlamydia-www.berkeley.edu:4231/, with the sequences described in [7], it was found that a family of 21 genes had the capacity to encode proteins belonging to this family. The presence of repeats of the amino acids GGAI was a common motif found in these proteins, and it is therefore suggested that they should be named GGAI proteins or Pmp proteins [11]. Most of the genes are clustered at two regions at the genome. It is surprising that a microorganism with a relatively small genome (1.23 mill base pairs) uses approximately 5.5 % of its coding capacity to encode these proteins. At both DNA and amino acid level the homology between the genes is quite low. The structure of the putative proteins is, however, similar with the repeated motif, GGAI, as the prevailing characteristic. The deduced amino acid sequences are shown in Figure 1. The Omp4–15 genes were sequenced by us and were thus independently named Omp4–15 [7, 8]. The rest of the Pmp genes is taken from the *C. pneumoniae* genome [10].

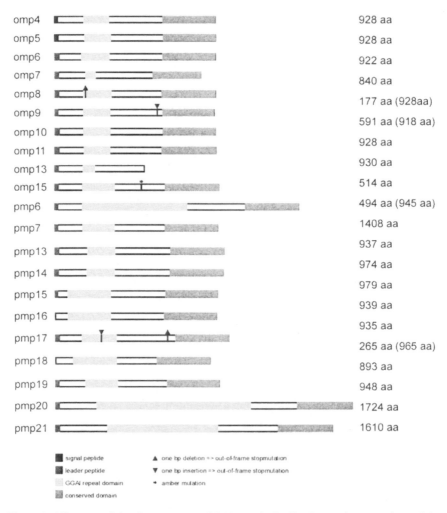

Figure 1. Alignment of the *C. pneumoniae* GGAI protein family. Comparison was done of the deduced amino acid sequences of the 21 *C. pneumoniae* GGAI proteins. The omp4–15 genes were sequenced by Knudsen et al. [7, and unpublished results], the pmp 1–21 genes were from the *C. pneumoniae* genomic sequence [10].

Two of the proteins have a cleavage site for signal peptidase 2 and are thus potential lipoproteins. Seventeen of the putative proteins have a cleavage site for signal peptidase 1 and are thus potential outer membrane proteins. Only two putative proteins have no leader sequence and thus do not have the capacity to migrate through the periplasmic membrane. In four of the genes a premature Stop codon occurs due to either a point mutation or an insertion or deletion of one nucleotide. One gene is seen as a short version. Structure prediction of the C-terminal part of the proteins shows that it is rich of beta-strands.

Migration of GGAI proteins in SDS-PAGE

Migration of Omp4 and Omp5 was studied by immunoblotting of purified *C. pneumoniae* EBs using antibodies against recombinant Omp4 and Omp5 (Figure 2). As shown [7, 8], the denatured GGAI proteins Omp4 and Omp5 migrate according to the predicted molecular size of 97–99 kDa (Figure 2A, lanes 1 and 2). Without boiling these proteins migrate much faster with a migration of approximately 70 kDa (Figure 2B, lanes 1 and 2). The reaction with the Omp5 antibody is identical to the reaction with the monoclonal antibody MAb 26.1 that binds to the surface of *C. pneumoniae* [12] (Figure 2B, lane 3).

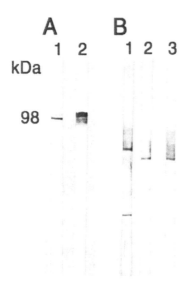

Figure 2. Immunological identification of Omp4 and Omp5 by immunoblotting. Purified *C. pneumoniae* EB proteins were separated by SDS-PAGE after boiling of the sample (A) or without boiling (B) and reacted with a polyclonal antibody against recombinant Omp4 and Omp5 (lanes 1 and 2, respectively) and with MAb 26.1 [6].

Antigenicity of GGAI proteins

In order to analyze the humoral immune response to infections caused by *C. pneumoniae*, four C57 black mice were intranasally infected with 10^7 *C. pneumoniae* inclusion forming units. Serum was obtained after 14 days. The serum samples were analyzed by immunoblotting with purified *C. pneumoniae* elementary bodies (EBs) as antigen [6]. When the antigen was boiled prior to separation of the proteins by SDS-PAGE, two of the four sera reacted strongly with the 60 kDa cysteine-rich outer membrane protein Omp2. The two other sera reacted only weakly with bands of different sizes. Without boiling prior to separation of the EB proteins by SDS-PAGE, all four sera reacted strongly with a band of approximately 70 kDa, presumably the GGAI proteins. This pattern of reaction indicates that during infection a strong antibody response is generated to conformational epitopes at the GGAI proteins but not to linear epitopes, as no antibody response was seen to a 98 kDa protein band in the SDS-PAGE of boiled EBs.

To analyze whether the Omp4 and 5 antigens were expressed during infection, mice lungs were examined by immunohistochemistry staining three days after infection. Rabbit polyclonal antibodies obtained by immunization of rabbits with purified recombinant Omp4 and 5 were used as antibodies for the staining. Both antibodies showed strong reaction with *C. pneumoniae* inclusion localized predominantly in the bronchial epithelial cells in parts of the lungs that showed heavy inflammation [12]. Thus both proteins seem to be expressed during infection of mice.

Immunoblotting with human sera

For many microorganisms immunoblotting has been useful for determination of the most immunogenic proteins. For *C. pneumoniae*, however, this has not been the case. When patient sera that were shown to be positive in the only species-specific sero-diagnostic test, the micro-immunofluorescence test (microIF), were analyzed in immunoblotting with purified EBs as antigen, a heterogeneous picture was seen [13-16]. Predominant protein bands differed from analysis to analysis but the overall impression was that only rarely Momp was recognized by the human humoral immune response. In these studies bands of 54 kDa and 98 kDa were frequently observed. To analyze whether differently prepared antigens would give a more homogeneous picture, we performed immunoblotting with 10 human serum samples of which 7 were shown to be positive by microIF and three as negative. As reference serum we used pAbdOmc. As antigens purified *C. pneumoniae* EBs were used without boiling prior to separation by SDS-PAGE (Figure 3A) and after boiling (Figure 3B). Reactions with the reference serum are shown in lanes 11. With unboiled EBs (Figure 3A, lane 11) the pAbdOmc reacted with three bands of which the strongest is migrating as Omp4–5. The other bands may contain other GGAI proteins. In lanes 3, 6 and 8 microIF-negative sera were investigated. No bands were seen. The microIF-positive sera all reacted differently, but most sera recognized bands with migration patterns as seen for the reference serum (4 of 7 with the lower band, 5 of 7 with the intermediate band and 3 of 7 with the highest band). In addition, several other bands could be observed. There was thus not a specific band that was recognized by all microIF-positive human sera. In Figure 3B the antigen was boiled prior to separation of the proteins by SDS-PAGE. The reference serum in lane 11 reacts, as expected, with Momp (39 kDa), Omp2 (60 kDa), a 75 kDa protein and the 97–99 kDa doublet band containing Omp4 [7]. As seen from the reactivity with microIF-positive sera, a heterogeneous reactivity pattern was observed in agreement with previous observations. All sera reacted weakly with the 97–99 kDa bands and with Momp, but since also the microIF-negative sera reacted, this could indicate that also the 97–99 kDa proteins may bind immunoglobulin as is known for Momp.

MicroIF is still the only species-specific sero-diagnostic test available. The complicated band pattern observed in immunoblotting even when not completely denatured proteins were used as antigen (Figure 3A) indicates a complex immune response. With our current knowledge that *C. pneumoniae* contains 21 GGAI proteins, of which different proteins may be expressed under infection, the complexity of reactivity of human serum samples could be high.

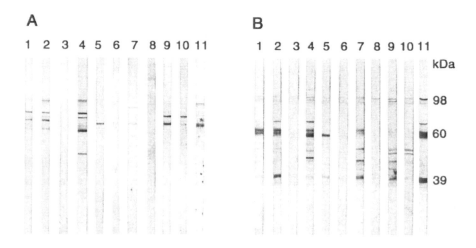

Figure 3. Immunoblotting of purified *C. pneumoniae* EB proteins separated by SDS-PAGE without boiling (A) or with boiling (B) of the samples. The separated proteins were transferred to nitrocellulose membranes that were cut in strips and reacted with human serum samples diluted 1:200 (lanes 1–10) and with a polyclonal antibody raised against SDS denatured *C. pneumoniae* OMC (7), lanes 11. Sera used in lanes 3, 6 and 8 were negative in the microIF test while the other sera were positive.

Conclusion and considerations for future work

The discovery of a novel proteinaceous layer on *C. pneumoniae* that contains only conformational epitopes can explain why progress in analysis of the pathogenicity has been so difficult. It raises the question whether such layers are found also on other pathogenic microorganisms. Furthermore, the identification of the novel surface layer will likely increase the development of diagnostic tests, and thus increase our understanding of its role in the development of acute and chronic diseases and their prevention. A prerequisite for that will be the ability to prepare recombinant proteins with a structure that can be recognized by antibodies present in human sera. Such correctly folded recombinant proteins would also be prerequisites for the analysis of protection and thus be potential vaccine candidates.

This novel, highly immunogenic surface layer may thus facilitate the development of a species-specific diagnostic test, and help determine the pathogenicity of this microorganism in acute and chronic diseases.

References

1. Caldwell HD, Schachter J (1982) Antigenic analysis of the major outer membrane protein of Chlamydia spp. Infect Immun 35: 1024–1031
2. Campbell LA, Kuo CC, Grayston JT (1990) Structural and antigenic analysis of *Chlamydia pneumoniae*. Infect Immun 58: 93–97
3. Grayston JT, Kuo CC, Wang S, Altman J (1986) A new *Chlamydia psittaci* strain, TWAR, isolated in acute respiratory tract infections. N Engl J Med 315: 161–168
4. Kuo CC, Grayston JT, Campbell LA, Goo YA, Wissler RW, Benditt EP (1995) *Chlamydia pneumoniae* (TWAR) in coronary arteries of young adults (15–34 years old). Proc Natl Acad Sci USA 92: 6911–6914
5. Jackson LA, Campbell LA, Kuo CC, Rodrigues DI, Lee A, Grayston JT (1997) Isolation of *Chlamydia pneumoniae* from a carotid endarterectomy specimen. J Infect Dis 176: 292–295
6. Christiansen G, Ostergaard L, Birkelund S (1997) Molecular biology of the *Chlamydia pneumoniae* surface. Scand J Infect Dis Suppl 104: 5–10
7. Knudsen K, Madsen AS, Mygind P, Christiansen G, Birkelund S (1999) Identification of two novel genes encoding 97- to 99-kilodalton outer membrane proteins of *Chlamydia pneumoniae*. Infect Immun 67: 375–383
8. Knudsen K, Madsen AS, Mygind P, Christiansen G, Birkelund S (1998) In: Stephens RS, Byrne GI, Christiansen G, Clarke IN, Grayston JT, Rank RG, Ridgway GL, Saikku P, Schachter J, Stamm WE (eds) Chlamydia infections. Proceedings of the Ninth International Symposium on Human Chlamydia Infections. University of California, San Francisco, pp 267–270
9. Melgosa MP, Kuo CC, Campbell LA (1993) Outer membrane complex proteins of *Chlamydia pneumoniae*. FEMS Microbiol Lett 112: 199–204
10. Stephens R: http://chlamydia-www.berkeley.edu:4231
11. Grimwood J, Mitchell W, Stephens RS (1998) In: Stephens RS, Byrne GI, Christiansen G, Clarke IN, Grayston JT, Rank RG, Ridgway GL, Saikku P, Schachter J, Stamm WE (eds) Chlamydia infections. Proceedings of the Ninth International Symposium on Human Chlamydia Infections. University of California, San Francisco, pp 263–266
12. Birkelund S, Knudsen K, Madsen AS, Falk E, Mygind P, Christiansen G (1998) In: Stephens RS, Byrne GI, Christiansen G, Clarke IN, Grayston JT, Rank RG, Ridgway GL, Saikku P, Schachter J, Stamm WE (eds) Chlamydia infections. Proceedings of the Ninth International Symposium on Human Chlamydia Infections. University of California, San Francisco, pp 275–278
13. Campbell LA, Kuo CC, Wang SP, Grayston JT (1990) Serological response to *Chlamydia pneumoniae* infection. J Clin Microbiol 28: 1261–1264
14. Iijima Y, Miyashita N, Kishimoto T, Kanamoto Y, Soejima R, Matsumoto A (1994) Characterization of *Chlamydia pneumoniae* species-specific proteins immunodominant in humans. J Clin Microbiol 32: 583–588

15. Jantos CA, Heck S, Roggendorf R, Sen-Gupta M, Heegemann J (1997) Antigenic and molecular analyses of different *Chlamydia pneumoniae* strains. J Clin Microbiol 35: 620–623
16. Kutlin A, Roblin PM, Hammerschlag MR (1998) Antibody response to *Chlamydia pneumoniae* infection in children with respiratory illness. J Infect Dis 177: 720–724

Discussion

Brade:

Dr. Christiansen, you said at the beginning that *C. pneumoniae* is not trafficking along acting filaments like *C. trachomatis* does, and accordingly you see these multiple inclusions in cells. But in the slide you showed from your animal models these were fantastic inclusions as they are known from *C. trachomatis*. I have rarely seen such inclusions with *C. pneumoniae*. Would you not consider that perhaps under *in vivo* situations *C. pneumoniae* may be trafficking as well along acting filaments because the *in vitro* culture of *C. pneumoniae* is so artificial? Even for *C. trachomatis* the *in vitro* culture is artificial, so that perhaps they are using the same routes.

Christiansen:

Yes, you are right. When you use an artificial system like cell culture where you even stop the protein synthesis in the host cells, it is a completely different situation. Still, that was what we could compare from *C. trachomatis* to *C. pneumoniae*, the same type of cell cultures. However, you are correct that the *in vivo* situation where you have an infection of the lungs may be totally different.

Yes, the inclusions look as if they were much more gathered in one cell. It is difficult to see, because the sections we have used here are quite thin, whether the inclusions are higher up or further down in the cytoplasm.

Brade:

Did you study the phosphorylation in the *in vivo* model?

Christiansen:

It will probably be difficult but of course we could try. We have to use much earlier time points, but first you have to identify the Chlamydia and then also look for the phosphorylation. But maybe by using some more natural cell lines it could be studied.

Chapter 2
Diagnosis of *Chlamydia pneumoniae* Infections

2.1
Direct detection of *Chlamydia pneumoniae* in atherosclerotic plaques

M. Maass

Introduction

Chlamydia pneumoniae has recently been established as a third species of the obligate intracellular Chlamydiae. Respiratory epithelium was identified as its primary target and the pathogen is now recognized as an important cause of mild community-acquired pneumonia, pharyngitis, and bronchitis [5, 8, 12]. *C. pneumoniae* is characterized by an extraordinarily high seroprevalence: seroepidemiological surveys indicate virtually everybody to be infected with the organism at least once during lifetime and reinfections to be common [12]. Nevertheless, it has been extremely difficult to recover viable isolates from the site of infection. In fact, this difficulty in adapting primary isolates to the artificial conditions of cell culture has been the reason why this extremely frequent bacterial pathogen has not been identified earlier than 1986 [8]. As chlamydiae are quite notorious for causing persistent disease with severe tissue destruction, concern on sequelae from recurrent chlamydial infection is justified [32]. In this respect, coronary artery disease has been related to prior or persistent *C. pneumoniae* infection [28-30]. Based on antichlamydial IgG elevation and the presence of immune complexes containing chlamydial lipopolysaccharide in coronary heart disease patients, *C. pneumoniae* infection was suggested as an independent cardiovascular risk factor in studies from Finland [28, 29]. These results proved reproducible wherever the attempt was made [18, 22, 31]. However, these indirect statistical associations cannot provide evidence of causality.

Endovascular infection might provide an explanation for yet unclear phenomena of atherogenesis like mesenchymal cell proliferation and the distinct inflammatory component [14]. A contribution of *C. pneumoniae* in this respect requires its presence in diseased arteries, and several investigators now have reported an occurrence of pathogen-specific structures like lipopolysaccharide epitopes and segments of genomic DNA in atheromatous plaques, though detection rates varied widely with the techniques employed. In fact, reported endovascular occurrence of *C. pneumoniae* has varied from 2 to 79 % in larger studies [4, 23, 33]. The actual rate of vessels potentially infected and the distribution of the organism in the vascular system is thus unknown. If a chlamydial occurrence in atheromatous plaques

Table 1: Direct detection results for *Chlamydia pneumoniae* in atherosclerotic lesions vary with the techniques used

Origin of vascular sample	Direct detection method	Positivity rate	Geographical region	Reference
Atherosclerotic coronary artery	Immunofluorescence	79 %	USA	(23)
	Immunohistochemistry	39 %	USA	(11)
	Immunohistochemistry	45 %	Japan	(26)
	Immunohistochemistry	42 %	South Africa	(13)
	Immunohistochemistry	45 %	USA	(4)
	Culture	8 %	USA	(27)
	Culture	0 %	USA	(33)
	Culture	16 %	Germany	(16)
	PCR	17 %	USA	(11)
	PCR	55 %	Japan	(26)
	PCR	43 %	South Africa	(13)
	PCR	32 %	USA	(4)
	PCR	2 %	USA	(33)
	PCR	26 %	Germany	(17)
Aortic valve	PCR	49 %	Sweden	(24)
Carotid artery	Immunohistochemistry	57 %	USA	(7)
	Immunohistochemistry	55 %	Japan	(35)
	Culture	6 %	USA	(9)
	PCR	15 %	Germany	(21)
Aorta	Immunohistochemistry	33 %	USA	(10)
	PCR	18 %	Germany	(17)
	PCR	44 %	UK	(25)
	PCR	51 %	Italy	(2)
A. iliaca	Immunohistochemistry	40 %	Japan	(26)
	PCR	55 %	UK	(25)
	PCR	30 %	Japan	(26)
	PCR	15 %	Germany	(17)

is indeed a newly recognized general phenomenon of atherosclerotic disease, examination of peripheral arteries prone to atherosclerosis will have to reproduce the presence of the pathogen, too. Recent studies have reported cultural recovery of *C. pneumoniae* from plaques and thus provided ultimate evidence of the presence of a bacterial organism in the chronic inflammatory process of atherosclerosis. This review will briefly summarize what has been achieved in detecting the fastidious obligate intracellular pathogen within atherosclerotic lesions.

Immunohistochemistry

Immunological staining has been widely applied to sections of atherosclerotic vessels in various stages of the disease. Positivity rates for chlamydial presence in atherosclerotic lesions usually vary between 33 % and 79 %; Table 1 gives an overview. Though interpretation of staining results is not easy and not always unequivocal, chlamydial structures appear to be present in endothelial and smooth muscle cells. Antibodies against chlamydial outer membrane proteins as well as against lipopolysaccharide components have been used in these studies. Though there is no standardization between laboratories, the results appear reproducible when carefully controlled. Positivity rates may be somewhat higher than in studies using PCR-based detection protocols, and one reason for this may be unexpected antibody reactivity or unspecific binding within the atherosclerotic lesions that expose distinctly altered lipid epitopes in comparison to healthy vessels [34]. With respect to the technique used and the positivity rates found, the study of Muhlestein et al. is remarkable [23]. In this study, immunofluorescence staining of coronary artery samples resulted in detection of *C. pneumoniae* in 79 % of cases. However, due to a strong autofluorescent activity in plaques and the resulting specificity problems, other groups have not yet been able to reproduce these findings.

PCR

PCR is meanwhile an established diagnostic method for *C. pneumoniae* infections that yields clinically relevant data as determined with respiratory specimens [5]. Detection of genomic DNA avoids the specificity problems potentially caused by altered tissue antigenicity in immunological detection protocols and thus should give more specific evidence for the presence of intact pathogen than detection of single epitopes. However, positivity rates have been more variable than found with immunohistochemistry and range in the larger studies between 2 % and 55 %; Table 1 gives an overview. The reason for this is apparently less one of regional variation than one of lack of standardization. Figure 1 lists some crucial points that apparently lead to the difficulties in obtaining comparable results. Two points appear especially noteworthy: First, using samples recovered during coronary angiography after rotational ablation and similar procedures results in negative or distinctly lower detection rates than otherwise seen with surgically removed vascular materials. Samples from catheter ablation are not satisfactory for the detection of vascular *C. pneumoniae* infection. Second, nested PCR appears to produce less positive results than classical PCR protocols. The nested PCR protocols are considered more specific than classical protocols as they contain an added DNA hybridization step. The different positivity rates may therefore indicate that classical PCR produces a greater number of false-positive results due to unspecific amplification products than nested protocols. The least standard to guarantee specificity of amplification products when using a classical PCR should be the subsequent use of a Southern Blot. For comparable results between laboratories the combined use of a nested PCR and a Southern Blot appears least prone to false-positive results. Using such a protocol, we have detected chlamydial presence as a generalized phenomenon of atherosclerosis in 26 % of vascular samples obtained at coronary revascularization procedures, in 15 % of samples from carotid endarterectomy, 18 % of aortic wall samples, and 15 % of A. iliaca samples, but not in 17 healthy control samples. Endovascular infection was restricted to macroscopically altered arterial tissue. Whether chlamydiae are homogeneously or focally distributed within the lesions is not known. In carotid atherectomy samples there was a tendency towards infection of progressed plaques [21]. *C. pneumoniae* can also be found in restenotic venous bypass grafts indicating infection subsequent to surgery [1, 17].

PCR-modification
- Classical PCR
- Nested PCR
- RT-rRNA PCR

PCR Primer Origin
- Pst I genomic DNA fragment
- 16S rRNA gene
- MOMP-gene/other defined genes

DNA–Extraction Method
- Digestion/heat
- Phenol/CTAB
- Solid phase

Sample Recovery/Treatment Method
- Surgical removal
- Catheter ablation
- Formalin-fixation

Figure 1. Parameters known to affect PCR.

At this moment, DNA detection appears as the most widely applicable technique to identify vascular chlamydial infection. A collaborative effort is urgently needed to provide an acceptable standardized diagnostic protocol for further research on vascular infection and atherogenesis. An ongoing attempt to compare PCR protocols from various laboratories may already provide some clarification on detection protocols (Jens Boman, personal communication). As we do not understand the possible mechanisms of chlamydial contribution to atherosclerosis, we do not know if DNA- or antigen-detection is a better indicator of pathogenetic relevance. DNA detection is a better method if viable bacteria are involved, antigen detection may be a better indicator if a deposit of undegraded chlamydial antigen triggers inflammatory responses within the vascular wall.

Cell Culture

Genomic DNA detection gives a good indication for the presence of intact viable pathogen as extrinsic DNA of dead bacteria is usually rapidly degraded by human restriction endonucleases. However, PCR cannot finally differentiate between replicating and non-replicating organisms. Therefore the final proof for the presence of viable bacteria – prerequisite for antimicrobial therapy – depends on positive culture results. In spite of the known difficulty in obtaining primary isolates of *C. pneumoniae*, several groups have attempted to recover the pathogen from homogenized atherosclerotic plaques. Meanwhile clear evidence exists that atheromata really harbor viable, culturally retrievable Chlamydia: several strains have been retrieved from plaques [9, 15, 27] (Table 1). Single isolates were reported from the carotid artery and the coronary artery [9, 27] in the USA. Using an optimized culture protocol [20], *C. pneumoniae* was recovered from 11/70 (16%) of coronary artery samples collected during surgical revascularization procedures in Germany [16]. Thus the presence of viable bacteria that are able to replicate in atherosclerotic plaques has been reproducibly demonstrated. The isolated strains appear to be susceptible to antichlamydial drugs [6]. However, the problems with cultural recovery of *C. pneumoniae* still result in a distinctly decreased sensitivity of even the most current culture procedures in comparison to PCR. Furthermore, presence of DNA in the absence of cultural recovery could be consistent with temporarily non-replicating bacteria causing persistent disease. Clearly, cultural attempts have been necessary to demonstrate the presence of viable bacteria within lesions and to recover vascular strains for further characterization, but laborious cell culture protocols involving eight and more subcultures are not the diagnostic assay of choice for identifying infected vessels.

Conclusion

The endovascular presence of genomic DNA of a pathogen generally susceptible to antimicrobial therapy in a substantial proportion of patients suffering from one of the major health hazards in industrialized countries can be of immense importance for public health. Pathogenesis research will focus on animal models, the inflammatory process within the plaque, the persistent state, and the genetics of the vascular isolates. However, it will be extremely difficult to apply research results to the patients. The crucial problem is that we are lacking a valid parameter to predict the risk of coronary artery infection in the individual. Diagnostic procedures like PCR that depend on coronary atherectomy samples are obviously too late in the course of the disease, and require standardization in a collaborative international effort. What we need is a reliable diagnostic assay based on peripheral blood. Surprisingly, serological results that once established the association are not useful in predicting the risk to harbor *C. pneumoniae* in the individual case. MIF-titers do not identify patients with vascular infection [19]. Better characterization of pathogenicity-related antigens and their production for diagnostic assays apparently is needed. But this again is extremely difficult, given the fact that the common molecular biological tools used in pathogenicity research do not apply to the intracellular chlamydiae. Lack of a valid diagnostic parameter for vascular infection also prevents any directed intervention in the patient. Recent studies indicate that circulating blood monocytes may carry chlamydial DNA [3]. The clinical relevance of this finding is not yet clear but may result in a better parameter to predict the vascular infection risk. Thus, apart from clinically controlled treatment studies, antimicrobial therapy in coronary artery disease patients is not yet justified. Unfortunately, the current large antimicrobial treatment trials do not appear to collect the materials, e.g., EDTA blood or PBMC fractions, that would be most helpful in establishing diagnostic tests and assessing their relevance.

The direct association between arteriosclerosis and a bacterial pathogen susceptible to antimicrobial treatment urgently requires further investigation. Current results imply a chlamydial role in the pathogenesis of coronary artery disease, but they are no final proof of a chlamydial etiology in atherogenesis. Thus, the occurrence of chlamydiae in a significant proportion of plaques is indicative of an infectious component in atherosclerosis, but whether chlamydiae actually initiate atherosclerotic injury, facilitate its progression, or merely colonize pre-existing lesions is unknown.

References

1. Bartels C, Maass M, Bein G, Malisius R, Brill N, Bechtel JFM, Sayk F, Feller AC, Sievers HH (1999) Detection of *Chlamydia pneumoniae* but not Cytomegalovirus in occluded saphenous vein coronary-artery bypass grafts. Circulation 99: 879–882
2. Blasi F, Denti F, Erba M, Cosentini R, Raccanelli R, Rinaldi A, Fragetti L, Esposito G, Ruberti U, Allegra L (1996) Detection of *Chlamydia pneumoniae* but not *Helicobacter pylori* in atherosclerotic plaques of aortic aneurysms. J Clin Microbiol 34: 2766–2769
3. Boman J, Soderberg S, Forsberg J, Birgander LS, Allard A, Persson K, Jidell E, Kumlin U, Juto P, Waldenstrom A (1998) High prevalence of *Chlamydia pneumoniae* DNA in peripheral blood mononuclear cells in patients with cardiovascular disease and in middle-aged blood donors. J Infect Dis 178: 274–277
4. Campbell LA, O'Brien ER, Cappuccio AL, Kuo CC, Wang SP, Stewart D, Patton DL, Cummings PK, Grayston JT (1995) Detection of *Chlamydia pneumoniae* TWAR in human coronary atherectomy tissues. J Infect Dis 172: 585–588
5. Dalhoff K, Maass M (1996) *Chlamydia pneumoniae* pneumonia in hospitalized patients: Clinical characteristics and diagnostic value of PCR detection in BAL. Chest 110: 351–356
6. Gieffers J, Solbach W, Maass M (1998) *In vitro* susceptibility of *Chlamydia pneumoniae* strains recovered from atherosclerotic coronary arteries. Antimicrob Agents Chemother 42: 2762–2764
7. Grayston JT, Kuo CC, Coulson AS, Campbell LA, Lawrence RD, Lee MJ, Strandness ED, Wang SP (1995) *Chlamydia pneumoniae* (TWAR) in atherosclerosis of the carotid artery. Circulation 92: 3397–3400
8. Grayston JT, Kuo CC, Wang SP, Altman J (1986) A new *Chlamydia psittaci* strain, TWAR, isolated in acute respiratory tract infections. N Engl J Med 315: 161–168
9. Jackson LA, Campbell LA, Kuo CC, Rodriguez DI, Lee A, Grayston JT (1997) Isolation of *Chlamydia pneumoniae* from a carotid endarterectomy specimen. J Infect Dis 176: 292–295

10. Kuo CC, Gown AM, Benditt EP, Grayston JT (1993) Detection of *Chlamydia pneumoniae* in aortic lesions of atherosclerosis by immunocytochemical stain. Arterioscler Thromb 13: 1501–1504
11. Kuo CC, Grayston JT, Campbell LA, Goo YA, Wissler RW, Benditt EP (1995) *Chlamydia pneumoniae* (TWAR) in coronary arteries of young adults (15–34 years old). Proc Natl Acad Sci USA 92: 6911–6914
12. Kuo CC, Jackson LA, Campbell LA, Grayston JT (1995) *Chlamydia pneumoniae* (TWAR). Clin Microbiol Rev 8: 451–461
13. Kuo CC, Shor A, Campbell LA, Fukushi H, Patton DL, Grayston JT (1993) Demonstration of *Chlamydia pneumoniae* in atherosclerotic lesions of coronary arteries. J Infect Dis 167: 841–849
14. Libby P (1996) Atheroma: more than mush. Lancet 348 (suppl I): s4–s7
15. Maass M (1996) *Chlamydia pneumoniae* in der Ätiologie respiratorischer und vaskulärer Erkrankungen des Menschen. Lübeck: Habilitationsschrift
16. Maass M, Bartels C, Engel PM, Mamat U, Sievers HH (1998) Endovascular presence of viable *Chlamydia pneumoniae* is a common phenomenon in coronary artery disease. J Am Coll Cardiol 31: 827–832
17. Maass M, Bartels C, Krüger S, Krause E, Engel PM, Dalhoff K (1998) Endovascular presence of *Chlamydia pneumoniae* is a generalized phenomenon in atherosclerotic vascular disease. Atherosclerosis 140: S25–S30
18. Maass M, Gieffers J (1996) Prominent serological response to *Chlamydia pneumoniae* in cardiovascular disease. Immunol Infect Dis 6: 65–70
19. Maass M, Gieffers J, Krause E, Engel PM, Bartels C, Solbach W (1998) Poor correlation between microimmunofluorescence serology and polymerase chain reaction results for detection of vascular *C. pneumoniae* infection in coronary artery disease patients. Med Microbiol Immunol 187: 103–106
20. Maass M, Harig U (1995) Evaluation of culture conditions used for isolation of *Chlamydia pneumoniae*. Am J Clin Pathol 103: 141–148
21. Maass M, Krause E, Engel PM, Krüger S (1997) Endovascular presence of *Chlamydia pneumoniae* in patients with hemodynamically effective carotid artery stenosis. Angiology 48: 699–706
22. Mendall MA, Carrington D, Strachan D, Patel P, Molineaux N, Levi J, Toosey T, Camm AJ, Northfield TC (1995) *Chlamydia pneumoniae*: risk factors for seropositivity and association with coronary heart disease. J Infect 30: 121–128
23. Muhlestein JB, Hammond EH, Carlquist JF, Radicke E, Thomson MJ, Karagounis LA, Woods ML, Anderson JL (1996) Increased incidence of Chlamydia species within the coronary arteries of patients with symptomatic atherosclerotic versus other forms of cardiovascular disease. J Am Coll Cardiol 27: 1555–1561
24. Nystrom-Rosander C, Thelin S, Hjelm E, Lindquist O, Pahlson C, Friman G (1997) High incidence of *Chlamydia pneumoniae* in sclerotic heart valves of patients undergoing aortic valve replacement. Scand J Infect Dis 29: 361–365
25. Ong G, Thomas BJ, Mansfield AO, Davidson BR, Taylor-Robinson D (1996) Detection and widespread distribution of *Chlamydia pneumoniae* in the vascular system and its possible implications. J Clin Pathol 49: 102–106

26. Ouchi K, Fujii B, Kanamoto Y, Karita M, Shirai M, Nakazawa T (1998) *Chlamydia pneumoniae* in coronary and iliac arteries of Japanese patients with atherosclerotic cardiovascular diseases. J Med Microbiol 47: 907–913
27. Ramirez JA, *Chlamydia pneumoniae*/Atherosclerosis Study Group (1996) Isolation of *Chlamydia pneumoniae* from the coronary artery of a patient with coronary arteriosclerosis. Ann Intern Med 125: 979–982
28. Saikku P, Leinonen M, Mattila K, Ekman MR, Nieminen MS, Mäkelä PH, Huttunen JK, Valtonen V (1988) Serological evidence of an association of a novel Chlamydia, TWAR, with chronic coronary heart disease and acute myocardial infarction. Lancet ii: 983–986
29. Saikku P, Leinonen M, Tenkanen L, Linnanmäki E, Ekman MR, Manninen V, Mänttäri M, Frick MH, Huttunen JK (1992) Chronic *Chlamydia pneumoniae* infection as a risk factor for coronary heart disease in the Helsinki Heart study. Ann Intern Med 116: 273–278
30. Thom DH, Grayston JT, Siscovick DS, Wang SP, Weiss NS, Daling JR (1992) Association of prior infection with *Chlamydia pneumoniae* and angiographically demonstrated coronary artery disease. JAMA 268: 68–72
31. Thom DH, Wang SP, Grayston JT (1991) *Chlamydia pneumoniae* strain TWAR antibody and angiographically demonstrated coronary artery disease. Arterioscler Thromb 11: 547–551
32. Ward ME (1995) The immunobiology and immunopathology of chlamydial infections. APMIS 103: 769–796
33. Weiss SM, Roblin PM, Gaydos CA, Cummings PK, Patton DL, Schulhoff N, Shani J, Frankel R, Penney K, Quinn TC, Hammerschlag MR, Schachter J (1996) Failure to detect *Chlamydia pneumoniae* in coronary atheromas of patients undergoing atherectomy. J Infect Dis 173: 957–962
34. Wissler RW (1995) Significance of *Chlamydia pneumoniae* (TWAR) in atherosclerotic lesions [editorial]. Circulation 92: 3376
35. Yamashita K, Ouchi K, Shirai M, Gondo T, Nakazawa T, Ito H (1998) Distribution of *Chlamydia pneumoniae* infection in the atherosclerotic carotid artery. Stroke 29: 773–778

Discussion

Brade:

I have to repeat a comment, Dr. Maass, although I made it already several times. When you are using the LPS antibodies in immunohistology, the audience should not believe that these could be false-positive reactions due to unspecificity. These are not antibodies directed against the lipid component, they are directed against the saccharide, they are not sticking to the plaques. If you get higher positivity with an LPS antibody in these studies instead of using a *C. pneumoniae* antibody, the conclusion should be that there are other chlamydial species which are also able to go into the arterial cell wall and not to say that there could be a cross reactivity with lipids.

Maass:

I leave that as a comment.

Klos:

Atherosclerosis is a chronic disease. If you search for Chlamydia by PCR or by culture, one would expect that you would find Chlamydia more often if you did this repeatedly. If you have a certain percentage of the population which is infected only by the acute disease, maybe 10 %, it might be that this is only the case for about two weeks. So if you repeat the PCR (or the attempt to culture, which is too difficult), is it then easier to find a risk factor if the PCR is three times positive within three months or six months? Then it is more a chronic status. If it is only positive once, then it might be an acute infection and is no indication for an atherosclerotic disease.

Maass:

You are referring to the PBMC. Of course, we could not repetitively recover coronary artery samples from individual patients. However, for peripheral blood samples this is possible. We are conducting a therapeutic trial on the use of azithromycin in coronary artery disease patients. From those patients, blood samples are collected at defined intervals for six months and examined by several PCR methods and by culture. We will be able to look at these statistical issues soon. However, we still cannot differentiate acute from chronic infection by the current PCR protocols. We will perhaps be able to draw conclusions on viability if we see significant differences in the culture results among various defined patient groups, e.g., patients with restenosis of a bypass graft vs. patients with primary coronary arteriosclerosis. Then we may conclude that there appear to be replicative Chlamydia in this patient group and non-replicative Chlamydia in the other. As culture is very insensitive and a PCR targeted on DNA will not provide us with those urgently needed results, we are establishing an RT-PCR to detect chlamydial mRNA and thus the metabolically active pathogen. This may once help to answer the question of chlamydial viability.

2.2
Detection of *Chlamydia pneumoniae* DNA in white blood cells

J. Boman

To diagnose *C. pneumoniae*, we have to use different strategies depending on the type of infection (acute or chronic). For diagnosing acute primary infection and acute re-infection useful diagnostic means are available. The best combination seems to be serology by MIF in combination with detection of *C. pneumoniae* in the respiratory tract by PCR and/or cell culture. Since *C. pneumoniae* can persist in the respiratory tract [1], serology can be used to distinguish between an acute and a persistent infection.

Concerning diagnosis of chronic *C. pneumoniae* infections, the situation is more complicated. Serology is not very useful for identifying individuals carrying *C. pneumoniae* in the vascular wall [2]. Therefore, we need tools for identifying *C. pneumoniae* carriers and for assessing microbiologic efficacy in clinical trials. There are several important questions: How frequent are chronic infections? Who is infected? Is it like tuberculosis? Once you get *C. pneumoniae*, you might have the bacterium in your body for the rest of your life. Is it possible to prevent a chronic infection if you treat patients early in the acute phase? If you have a chronic infection, is it possible to eradicate the bacterium? Several antibiotic treatment trials of patients with coronary heart disease have started. Early results from some of them indicate that it may be quite complicated to eradicate *C. pneumoniae* using monotherapy with antibiotics if there are signs of chronic *C. pneumoniae* infection. For treating patients with a persistent infection, what is the optimum regimen? Monotherapy? Which antibiotic? Should we use a combination of antibiotics? Adding other agents, such as immunostimulating agents in combination with antibiotics? How long should we treat the patients? One year, one month, two weeks? Pulse therapy? At the moment, nobody knows. Perhaps *C. pneumoniae* can be activated and more susceptible to antibiotic therapy if the patients are pretreated with steroids?

So several important questions are addressed and to answer these we need better tools to identify individuals carrying *C. pneumoniae* and to monitor therapy. Maass et al. [3] have shown that the antibody level cannot be used to predict carriage of *C. pneumoniae* in the vessel wall, but there is a good correlation between a negative serology and a negative PCR. Maybe serology can be used as a screening tool to identify individuals at increased risk of carrying *C. pneumoniae*? But presence of antibodies doesn't tell you if there is an ongoing or a previous infection.

Culture is the gold standard. In acute infection, there seems to be a good agreement between culture, PCR and serology [4]. However, there is a problem diagnosing chronic infection: culture is not very sensitive, especially on vascular tissue or peripheral blood mononuclear cells (PBMCs). Thus, a negative culture does not exclude the presence of *C. pneumoniae.* PCR detection of *C. pneumoniae* DNA or mRNA may be a more useful means. By PCR, it may be possible to find evidence of the bacterium both in the vascular wall and in white blood cells. Similarly, some other intracellular bacteria can be found in macrophages and monocytes, e.g. *M. tuberculosis.* Condos et al. [5] showed that PBMCs can be used to identify individuals with an active TB infection: in this study from New York, 95 % of the patients with an active TB infection were positive by nested PCR in PBMCs. Also very important, the nPCR test on PBMCs could be used to monitor anti-TB therapy: within four months nearly all initially nPCR-positive patients on therapy reverted to negative.

Can a similar technique be used to detect *C. pneumoniae*? We analyzed by PCR vascular tissue from 40 patients with abdominal aortic aneurysms (AAA), a disease known to be associated with atherosclerosis, and tissue from 40 controls with normal aorta. *C. pneumoniae* DNA was significantly more frequently detected in AAA tissue compared with normal aortic tissue [6]. One question was: can serum be used for detection of *C. pneumoniae* DNA in patients who were positive in aortic tissue? Thirty-seven sera from these 40 patients with aneurysms were available. Unfortunately, only one serum sample was positive by nPCR (a serum sample from a tissue-positive patient). Thus, the sensitivity of serum PCR seemed to be low for identification of individuals carrying *C. pneumoniae* DNA in the vascular wall. PBMCs were collected from patients with coronary heart disease: 59 of 101 were repeatedly positive by nPCR. Healthy blood donors were used as controls: at the age of 40–45 years around 25 % were positive and an increasing prevalence by increasing age was found. In middle-aged and elderly there were similar rates as in patients with coronary heart disease (CHD) [7]. One-hundred-fifty negative PCR controls were included, all were negative. In parallel with PBMCs from CHD patients, PBMCs from young healthy blood donors aged 18 to 30 years were investigated. In this group, the prevalence of *C. pneumoniae* IgG antibodies was 67 %, but the prevalence of *C. pneumoniae* DNA was below 2 % (1/63). The prevalence of circulating Chlamydia-containing immune complexes in CHD patients and healthy controls seems to be similar to the prevalence of *C. pneumoniae* DNA found in PBMCs [8].

What does it mean to find *C. pneumoniae* DNA in PBMCs? In a study by Moazed et al. [9], it was shown that mice infected with *C. pneumoniae* were positive in PBMCs. The infection was active and could be transferred by PBMCs to uninfected mice. *C. pneumoniae* DNA was rapidly degraded and could not be used to infect uninfected mice if the cells were irradiated before transfer of the cells. This means it is very likely that carriage of *C. pneumoniae* DNA in PBMCs represents an ongoing *C. pneumoniae* infection.

Also, Maass et al. have shown that there is a good correlation between detection of viable *C. pneumoniae* in coronary arteries and detection of *C. pneumoniae* DNA in monocytes in peripheral blood [10].

For *C. pneumoniae* PCR, measuring chlamydial load can be done using the automated PRISM ABI 7700 PCR system. This test measures the PCR product after each PCR cycle. Using a standard curve it is then possible to calculate the copy number in the original samples. Unfortunately, the taq-polymerase used in the ABI PRISM 7700 system may not be the optimal enzyme for detection of *C. pneumoniae* DNA in PBMCs.

In conclusion, we need reliable tests for identifying carriers of *C. pneumoniae* and for monitoring therapy. *C. pneumoniae* PCR on PBMCs may be a useful tool for identifying carriers of *C. pneumoniae*, especially if a quantitative PCR is used.

References

1. Hammerschlag MR, Chirgwin K, Roblin PM, Gelling M, Dumornay W, Mandel L, Smith P, Schachter J (1992) Persistent infection with *Chlamydia pneumoniae* following acute respiratory illness. Clin Infect Dis 14: 178–182
2. Kuo CC, Shor A, Campbell LA, Fukushi H, Patton DL, Grayston JT (1993) Demonstration of *Chlamydia pneumoniae* in atherosclerotic lesions of coronary arteries. J Infect Dis 167: 841–849
3. Maass M, Gieffers J, Krause E, Engel PM, Bartels C, Solbach W (1998) Poor correlation between microimmunofluorescence serology and polymerase chain reaction for detection of vascular *Chlamydia pneumoniae* infection in coronary artery disease patients. Med Microbiol Immunol 187: 103–106
4. Boman J, Allard A, Persson K, Lundborg M, Juto P, Wadell G (1997) Rapid diagnosis of respiratory *Chlamydia pneumoniae* infection by nested touchdown polymerase chain reaction compared with culture and antigen detection by EIA. J Infect Dis 175: 1523–1526
5. Condos R, McClune A, Rom WN, Schluger NW (1996) Peripheral-blood-based PCR assay to identify patients with active pulmonary tuberculosis. Lancet 347: 1082–1085
6. Petersen E, Boman J, Persson K, Arnerlov C, Wadell G, Juto P, Eriksson A, Dahlen G, Angquist KA (1998) *Chlamydia pneumoniae* in human abdominal aortic aneurysms. Eur J Vasc Endovasc Surg 15: 138–142
7. Boman J, Soderberg S, Forsberg J, Birgander LS, Allard A, Persson K, Jidell E, Kumlin U, Juto P, Waldenstrom A, Wadell G (1998) High prevalence of *Chlamydia pneumoniae* DNA in peripheral blood mononuclear cells in patients with cardiovascular disease and in middle-aged blood donors. J Infect Dis 178: 274–277
8. Saikku P, Leinonen M, Tenkanen L, Linnanmäki E, Ekman MR, Manninen V, Manttari M, Frick MH, Huttunen JK (1992) Chronic *Chlamydia pneumoniae* infection as a risk factor for coronary heart disease in the Helsinki Heart Study. Ann Intern Med 116: 273–278
9. Moazed TC, Kuo CC, Grayston JT, Campbell LA (1998) Evidence of systemic dissemination of *Chlamydia pneumoniae* via macrophages in the mouse. J Infect Dis 177: 1322–1325
10. Maass M, Krause E, Kruger S, et al. (1997) Coronary arteries harbor viable *Chlamydia pneumoniae*. 8th European Congress of Clinical Microbiology and Infectious Diseases, Lausanne, Switzerland, May 25–28, 1997, abstract 578

Discussion

Ossewaarde:

I have a question on PCR results from peripheral mononuclear cells and vascular tissue. You told us that in both situations the percentage is almost the same. If you prepare your specimens from the vascular wall prior to PCR, you homogenize the specimen, including all the blood inside. So how do you know the Chlamydia is really inside the lesion and not in small blood vessels?

Boman:
We don't know that.

Ossewaarde:
So, in fact, you are correlating blood with blood.

Boman:
Yes, it could be so. But we also had a control group, vascular tissue from patients without atherosclerosis and we could rarely detect *C. pneumoniae* DNA in such normal vascular tissue. But you can have more cells, of course, in the inflamed atherosclerotic plaque, monocytes from the blood. We know that normal vascular tissue is PCR negative and atherosclerotic tissue is positive, but we do not know in which cells. It could be blood-derived mononuclear cells going in and out. I believe it is so.

Byrne:
Working with *C. pneumoniae* may be a lab safety issue situation, too. Have you looked at going from negative to positive in monocytes of any lab workers? Have you followed them to see if there really is a correlation between especially vascular wall colonization in monocyte positivity? Or does anyone have any information on that? Because that may be something we want to start thinking about.

Boman:
I am negative by serology and PCR. And the technicians working in our lab are all PCR negative in PBMCs. We wanted to do a pilot study in our lab but we couldn't find anyone positive.

Hammerschlag:
With anybody coming new into the lab, we routinely get a baseline serology and a nasal pharyngeal swab. So far, the only time we had a problem was when we had an exploding centrifuge with a flask scattered in the centrifuge, and two individuals got a nasal infection. Otherwise we had no documented seroconversions. One person probably was a community-acquired infection. We use the laminar flow for all work with *C. pneumoniae*.

Boman:
We routinely check the technicians by nasopharyngeal PCR just to see that they don't carry the bacterium for contamination reasons. We do that routinely as a control and they have all been negative. Otherwise they are not allowed to work in our lab with *C. pneumoniae* culture or PCR.

Cosentini:

Would you suggest an antibiotic treatment in patients with a coronary artery disease who are positive with your PCR in PBMC?

Boman:

Nobody knows at the moment if such individuals benefit from therapy. But there have been some treatment trials. If we look at other bacterial infections, e.g. *Helicobacter pylori*, the IgG and IgA antibodies will decline rapidly if the infection is eradicated. Regarding *C. pneumoniae*, in four treatment trials reported so far the antibodies were at stable high levels for at least six months in three of the studies. We have treated patients with macrolides and doxycycline and the titers were invariably high for months and years after therapy. It is not a proof but an indication that there is still an ongoing infection and no eradication. It might be very difficult to eradicate *C. pneumoniae* with monotherapy. Therefore we are planning to use combinations with other agents, not only antibiotics.

Saikku:

About these laboratory infections: we have seen two pneumonias in persons which were concentrating large amounts of *C. pneumoniae*. One was a very good example to follow how cell-mediated immunity against *C. pneumoniae* was developing.

Brade:

Just a brief comment on the persistence of antibody levels, I think that is also true for *C. trachomatis* infections. Even in cases where after antibiotic treatment the patients are without any clinical symptoms, there are cases which still have persisting high levels of IgA antibodies. We don't know whether these are silent persisting infections or whether this is persisting antigen.

Boman:

Yes, this has been shown in two studies from Norway. After treatment for one month using doxycycline, the *C. trachomatis* antibodies declined to undetectable levels within a few months. High stable levels that declined in the couples, both the males or females, were treated. So I also think this is true for *C. trachomatis* as well.

Anonymous:

Do you have any data on acute phase proteins or fibrinogen or other cardiovascular risk factors in patients who were PCR-positive compared with patients who were PCR-negative?

Boman:

We will do that in the planned treatment trial. We don't have the data yet, but we have included these parameters before, during and after therapy. There are many inflammatory markers that we want to measure.

Maass:

Regarding the possible persistence of *C. pneumoniae* in peripheral blood monocytes, could organ transplantation or a bone marrow transplantation transfer *C. pneumoniae* into the immunocompromised host? Should these donors be screened for *C. pneumoniae*?

Boman:

We are doing a study with recipients of blood from *C. pneumoniae*-positive donors. I don't have the results yet since the study is ongoing. It is a possibility based on mice studies in Seattle. On the other hand, most recipients are at least antibody positive.

2.3
Detection of *Chlamydia pneumoniae* in clinical specimens by PCR-EIA

C.A. Jantos

Chlamydia pneumoniae is an obligate intracellular bacterial pathogen and an important cause of respiratory tract infections in humans. Pneumonia and bronchitis are the most common clinical manifestations of *C. pneumoniae* infections. Approximately 10 % of cases of community-acquired pneumonia are associated with *C. pneumoniae*. In addition, there is growing evidence that the organism may play a role in atherogenesis, as several studies have demonstrated the presence of the organism in atherosclerotic lesions [8].

Laboratory methods for the diagnosis of *C. pneumoniae* infection include isolation of the organism in cell culture, serological assays, and DNA amplification tests. However, in contrast to *C. trachomatis*, *C. pneumoniae* is difficult to recover in cell cultures [7]. Serological diagnosis of *C. pneumoniae* infections is hampered by the slow antibody response to *C. pneumoniae*. Detection of a significant rise in antibody titers can take weeks and allows only a retrospective diagnosis. Furthermore, it has been demonstrated that some infected patients, especially children, do not develop an antibody response [1, 4].

PCR provides a more rapid alternative for the identification of *C. pneumoniae* infection. Numerous different single-step or nested PCR assays have been described in the literature for the molecular detection of the organism. The most common DNA targets used for the identification of the organism are the 16S rRNA gene, a specific PstI-DNA fragment and the major outer membrane protein gene (omp1) [2, 3, 9].

We have developed a rapid and simple PCR-EIA for the detection of *C. pneumoniae* [6]. Patient specimens such as throat swabs, BAL, sputum or atherectomy specimens are treated with proteinase K to release the DNA. The 16S rRNA gene is used as the target for amplification of *C. pneumoniae* DNA from clinical specimens. Primers CpnA and CpnB are used to amplify a 465-bp segment from the 16S rRNA gene of the organism. Primers CpnA and CpnF are used to generate a 446-bp internal probe, which is labeled by incorporation of digoxigenin during PCR. This probe is used for the detection of PCR products by an EIA.

In the first round of amplification samples are checked for the presence of inhibitory substances by using an internal control. Specimens which contain inhibitory substances are subjected to DNA extraction. In the second PCR, *C. pneumoniae* sequences are amplified from clinical specimens. All PCR reaction mixtures are treated with a heat-labile uracil-N-glycosylase (UNG) to control carryover contamination. PCR products generated from *C. pneumoniae* are detected by an EIA. After amplification and denaturation, the single stranded PCR product is hybridized to the DIG-labeled 446-bp probe. The resulting hybrid is bound to streptavidin-coated microtiter plates through the biotinylated primer

CpnB. Bound hybrids are then detected with anti-DIG peroxidase conjugate and a colorimetric substrate. The optical density of each specimen is determined with an EIA reader.

Under optimal conditions the sensitivity of this PCR-EIA is less than 1 inclusion forming unit or less than 10 elementary bodies of *C. pneumoniae*. The EIA for the detection of PCR products is nearly as sensitive as Southern blot analysis, but approximately 100 times more sensitive than the detection of PCR products by ethidium bromide staining of agarose gels.

Table 1. Comparison of cell culture and PCR-EIA for detection of *C. pneumoniae* in throat swab specimens[a].

Method	Nos. of clinical specimens with result	
	Positive	Negative
Cell culture	1	367
PCR-EIA	13	355

[a] from reference #6

In 368 throat swab specimens from children with respiratory tract infections we compared cell culture with the PCR-EIA for the detection of *C. pneumoniae*. Despite five passages of all specimens in cell cultures, the organism was isolated from only one of these samples. In contrast, 13 patient specimens were repeatedly positive by the PCR-EIA (Table 1). All these specimens could be confirmed as positive by an omp1-based nested PCR. This observation clearly demonstrates that PCR is superior to cell culture for the detection of the organism [6].

Table 2. Characteristics of CAD patients with evidence of *C. pneumoniae* infection[a].

Patient No.	sex/age	Coronary heart disease[b]	Risk factors	16S rRNA-PCR	omp1-PCR	MIF-IgG-titer
6	m/73	3 (R)	hy, li, dia	+	+	32
22	m/38	1	–	+	+	32
37	m/61	1 (R)	hy	–	+	ND
46	m/51	2	hy, li	–	+	–

[a] from reference #5
[b] 1 = one vessel disease; 2 = two vessel disease; 3 = three vessel disease; (R) = restenosis
CAD = coronary artery disease; dia = diabetes mellitus; hy = hypertension; li = hyperlipidemia; m = male; ND = not determined; + = positive in assay; – = negative in assay,

In another study we examined atherectomy specimens from 50 patients undergoing directional coronary atherectomy for the presence of *C. pneumoniae* by PCR [5]. *C. pneumoniae* DNA was detected by PCR in atherosclerotic plaques of four patients (8 %). Two patients' coronary atheromas were positive both by the

16S rRNA-based PCR-EIA and by an omp1-based nested PCR. The other two patients' specimens were positive only by the nested PCR (Table 2).

Various PCR procedures for the detection of *C. pneumoniae* by different detection systems are currently under investigation. However, these assays have not been compared with each other. Nested PCRs with omp1- or 16S rRNA-based primers have been reported to be more sensitive than single-step PCRs. In our study on the presence of *C. pneumoniae* in coronary atherectomy specimens, nested PCR turned out to be superior to the single-step PCR. However, a serious disadvantage of nested PCRs is the high risk of carryover contamination. In our hands nested PCR proved to be useful only as a confirmatory test but not for routine testing of clinical specimens. Furthermore, UNG which destroys PCR products from previous amplifications can be used in a nested PCR only in the second round of amplification.

Our PCR-EIA is the first PCR procedure described for the detection of *C. pneumoniae* which includes a dUTP-UNG system for carryover prevention. The EIA for the detection of PCR products is easy to perform and nearly as sensitive as Southern blotting.

All PCR-assays described so far in the literature are in-house PCRs. Since all these assays lack standardization, PCR results may vary among clinical microbiological laboratories. The lack of standardization of PCRs may account for the discrepancies between the results of different studies which examined the presence of *C. pneumoniae* in atherosclerotic lesions. Therefore, there is a need for the standardization of PCR assays. A commercially available DNA amplification test for the detection of *C. pneumoniae* would be an important advance in the field of diagnosis of *C. pneumoniae* infections.

References

1. Block S, Hedrick J, Hammerschlag MR, Cassell GH, Craft JC (1995) *Mycoplasma pneumoniae* and *Chlamydia pneumoniae* in pediatric community-acquired pneumonia: comparative efficacy and safety of clarithromycin vs. erythromycin ethylsuccinate. Pediatr Infect Dis J 14: 471–477
2. Campbell LA, Melgosa MP, Hamilton DJ, Kuo CC, Grayston JT (1992) Detection of *Chlamydia pneumoniae* by polymerase chain reaction. J Clin Microbiol 30: 434–439
3. Gaydos CA, Quinn TC, Eiden JJ (1992) Identification of *Chlamydia pneumoniae* by DNA amplification of the 16S rRNA gene. J Clin Microbiol 30: 796–800
4. Gaydos CA, Roblin PM, Hammerschlag MR, Hyman CL, Eiden JJ, Schachter J, Quinn TC (1994) Diagnostic utility of PCR-enzyme immunoassay, culture, and serology for detection of *Chlamydia pneumoniae* in symptomatic and asymptomatic patients. J Clin Microbiol 32: 903–905
5. Jantos CA, Nesseler A, Waass W, Baumgärtner W, Tillmanns H, Haberbosch W (1999) Low prevalence of *Chlamydia pneumoniae* in atherectomy specimens from patients with coronary heart disease. Clin Infect Dis 28: 988–992
6. Jantos CA, Roggendorf R, Wuppermann FN, Hegemann JH (1998) Rapid detection of *Chlamydia pneumoniae* by PCR-enzyme immunoassay. J Clin Microbiol 36: 1890–1894

7. Kuo CC, Grayston JT (1988) Factors affecting viability and growth in HeLa 229 cells of Chlamydia sp. strain TWAR. J Clin Microbiol 26: 812–815
8. Kuo CC, Jackson LA, Campbell LA, Grayston JT (1995) *Chlamydia pneumoniae* (TWAR). Clin Microbiol Rev 8: 451–461
9. Tong CY, Sillis M (1993) Detection of *Chlamydia pneumoniae* and *Chlamydia psittaci* in sputum samples by PCR. J Clin Pathol 46: 313–317

Discussion

Maass:

How are your arterectomy samples defined? Are they from coronary surgery or from catheter ablation?

Jantos:

These specimens are obtained by catheter ablation and are comparable to those specimens which have been examined by Weiss et al.

Maass:

The point is, people who use this kind of specimens find 2 % or 4 % positives. Using samples obtained at coronary surgery, they find 30 %. So the difference may be caused by the samples used.

Jantos:

The same type of samples have been examined by Jackson and by Muhlestein. In the same type of specimens both have found higher percentages of *C. pneumoniae*. However, Weiss has not. His results are comparable to our results. But these samples are very small and we cannot exclude that sample bias had an influence on our results.

Byrne:

I agree that we need a commercial standardized test. Does anybody here have any information about something like this on the horizon?

Jantos:

I don't. I wanted to point out that it would be a significant improvement. A reliable commercial diagnostic test would be a significant improvement in the field, not only for diagnosis but also to judge the results of many clinical studies. PCR results are not comparable between many laboratories.

Bhakdi:

As I recall, the Homburg/Saar group have also failed to find significant positivity for *C. pneumoniae* in their samples using a very good PCR.

2.4
State of the art in the diagnosis of acute and chronic *Chlamydia pneumoniae* infection

M.R. Hammerschlag

As *Chlamydia pneumoniae* is an obligate intracellular parasite capable of causing prolonged, often subclinical infection, diagnosis of *C. pneumoniae* infection is somewhat complicated. Although isolation of the organism implies infection, it may not imply that the organism is causing pneumonia or other respiratory infection in the patient. It is also unclear whether colonization or asymptomatic infection without disease elicits an antibody response. Multiple diagnostic methods have been evaluated, but there is no "gold standard" for determining whether disease occurring in an individual is due to *C. pneumoniae*. Although it has been suggested that there are differences in the antibody response to primary infection, reinfection and reactivated infection, there are limited data correlating serology with culture. This is further complicated by the lack of standardized methods for serology and nonculture methods such as polymerase chain reaction (PCR).

Culture of *C. pneumoniae*

C. pneumoniae can be isolated from nasopharyngeal (NP) and throat swabs, sputum and pleural fluid of patients with pneumonia, bronchitis and asthma [1, 3, 10, 13]. *C. pneumoniae* has also been isolated from middle ear fluids of children with acute otitis media [4]. The nasopharynx appears to be the optimum site for isolation of the organism, especially in children [3]. The relative yield from sputum is not known.

Initial studies suggested that *C. pneumoniae* was very difficult to isolate in tissue culture as compared with *C. trachomatis* [13]. Originally the same methods were used, HeLa or McCoy cells pretreated with dextran diethyl-aminiethyl (DEAE). Multiple passages were needed, the inclusions were very small and difficult to see and in general the yield was very poor. *C. pneumoniae* grows more readily in other cell lines derived from respiratory tissue, specifically HEp-2 and HL cells [8, 33, 37]. Omission of pretreatment with dextran DEAE results in much larger inclusions and specimens need only be passed once [32]. Culture with an initial inoculation and one passage should take 4 to 7 days. NP specimens for culture can be obtained with Dacron-tipped wire shafted swabs. Each lot of swabs should be tested in mock infection system as the adhesive used can be different from lot to lot, some adhesives can be inhibitory to growth of Chlamydia or toxic to the cells. Specimens for culture should be placed in appropriate transport media, usually a sucrose-phosphate buffer with antibiotics and fetal calf serum, and stored immediately at –70 °C. Viability decreases if specimens are held at room temperature. After 72 hours incubation, culture confirmation can be performed by staining with either a *C. pneumoniae* species-specific or a *Chlamydia* genus-specific (anti-LPS) fluorescein-conjugated monoclonal antibody [26]. There are no commercially produced *C. pneumoniae*-specific reagents available in the United States. Performance of these reagents has not been extensively evaluated. Studies suggest that staining characteristics can vary depending on strain of the organism and method of fixation [26, 35]. If a genus-specific antibody is used, *C. pneumoniae* should be confirmed by differential staining with a specific *C. trachomatis* antibody; if the latter is negative, then the isolate is either *C. pneumoniae* or *C. psittaci*. If there was no avian exposure, psittacosis would be highly unlikely.

Detection of antibody to *C. pneumoniae* in serum

The microimmunofluorescence (MIF) test

As isolation of *C. pneumoniae* was difficult and initially limited, initial emphasis was placed on serologic diagnosis. Grayston and colleagues proposed a set of criteria for serologic diagnosis of *C. pneumoniae* infection with the microimmunofluorescence (MIF) test that is used by many laboratories and clinicians [13]. For acute infection the patient should have a four-fold rise in IgG titer, a single IgM titer of 1:16 or greater, or a single IgG titer of 1:512 or higher. Past or pre-existing infection is defined as an IgG titer of 1:16 or higher but less than 1:512. It was further proposed that the pattern of antibody response in primary infection differed from that seen in reinfection [5]. In initial infection, the IgM response appears about 3 weeks after the onset of illness and the IgG response appears at 6 to 8 weeks. In reinfection, the IgM response may be absent and the IgG occurs earlier, within 1 to 2 weeks. Recently several investigators have proposed the use of IgA antibody as an indicator of chronic infection with *C. pneumoniae*. The rationale behind this is that the half-life of IgA is less than one week and that its continuous presence may indicate persistent antigenic stimulation. However, there are no criteria for IgA that have been correlated with culture, and different studies have used different cut-offs ranging from 1:8 to $\leq$ 1:256. We tested two patients with culture-documented chronic *C. pneumoniae* respiratory infection (periods up to 9 years); one had detectable anti-*C. pneumoniae* IgA by MIF ($\geq$ 1:16), the other did not [9].

Because of the relatively long period until the development of a serologic response in primary infection, the antibody response may be missed if convalescent sera are obtained too soon, i.e., earlier than 3 weeks after the onset of illness. Use of paired sera also only affords a retrospective diagnosis, which is of little help in terms of deciding how to treat the patient. The criteria for use of a single serum sample have not been correlated with the results of culture and are based mainly on data from adults. The antibody response in acute infection may take longer than 3 months to develop. Acute, culture-documented infection can also occur without seroconversion, especially in children. The correlation of culture and serology in three pneumonia treatment studies is summarized in table 1. As part of a multicenter pneumonia treatment study in children 3 through 12 years of age, Block et al. isolated *C. pneumoniae* from 34 of 260 (13.1 %) of the children enrolled. Serologic evidence of acute infection was found in 48 (18.5 %), but only

8 (23 %) of the culture-positive children met the serologic criteria for acute infection, most had no detectable antibody by the MIF test even after 3 months of follow up [3]. The majority of the "positive" serologic results in the culture-negative children were stable high IgG titers ($\geq$ 1:512). Seroconversions were infrequent. None of the children had detectable CF antibody. Similar results were reported in another pediatric pneumonia treatment study by Harris et al., only 5 (16 %) of 31 culture-positive children met the serologic criteria for acute infection [17]. The children in this multicenter study were 6 months through 16 years of age, the isolation rate of *C. pneumoniae* was 7.8 %. In another study in children, *C. pneumoniae* was isolated from 13 of 118 (11 %) children 5 to 15 years of age who were initially evaluated for either new or acute exacerbations of asthma [10]. Only 5 of the children with culture-confirmed infection had detectable IgG antibody to *C. pneumoniae*. One child who was noncompliant with his antibiotic therapy was culture-positive on five occasions over a 3-month period, but no anti-*C. pneumoniae* antibody was present at any time.

Table 1. Correlation of *C. pneumoniae* serology and culture in pneumonia treatment studies

study (ref #)	age range	n	Positive test for *C. pneumoniae*		
			culture	serology[a]	culture and serology
Block et al. [3]	3–12 y.o.	260	34 (13 %)	48 (18 %)	8 (3 %)
Harris et al. [17]	6 m–16 y.o.	456	31 (6.7 %)	32 (7 %)	5 (1.1 %)
Hammerschlag et al. [16]	12–93 y.o.	48	10 (20.8 %)	11 (23 %)	6 (12.5 %)

[a] 4-fold rise in specific IgG or IgM
Single IgM $\geq$ 1:16, or single IgG $\geq$ 1:512

When sera from culture-positive, but MIF-negative children with respiratory infection were examined by immunoblotting, over 89 % of these children had antibody to a number of *C. pneumoniae* proteins but only 24 % reacted with the major outer membrane protein (MOMP) [23]. These results were similar to those reported by others using sera from adults [2, 19, 20]. The MOMP does not appear to be immunodominant in the immune response to *C. pneumoniae* infection [30]. The MOMP is the major surface-exposed antigen of *C. trachomatis* and may be the major antigen in the MIF assay. The lack of reactivity in the MIF assay observed in children may be secondary to the lack of reactivity to the MOMP. Unfortunately, there was no reactivity to any *C. pneumoniae* protein or combination of proteins that could readily differentiate infected from uninfected children. When paired sera were examined, the band patterns remained the same for over 70 % of the children. In the remaining children, changes in the immunoblots of acute phase sera compared with convalescent sera were unique for each patient. When the same sera were immunoblotted against recent clinical isolates of *C. pneumoniae*, there were differences in the intensity of reaction and the band patterns, indicating possible antigenic diversity between the isolates. This has also been observed by other investigators with sera from adults [2, 19].

The correlation between culture and serology is higher in adults, but culture-documented infection in adults with pneumonia can also occur in the absence of seroconversion or detectable antibody by MIF [16] (Table 1). Background rates of seropositivity can also be very high in some adult populations. As part of a study of asymptomatic *C. pneumoniae* infection among subjectively healthy adults in Brooklyn, New York, Hyman et al. found 81 % to have IgG or IgM titers of 1:16 or greater [18]. Seventeen percent had evidence of "acute infection", IgG equal or greater than 1:512 and/or IgM equal or greater than 1:16. However, none of these individuals were culture- or PCR-positive. Similar results were reported by Kern et al. among healthy firefighters and policemen in Rhode Island [22]. The specificity of the MIF IgM assay can be affected by the presence of rheumatoid factor. A study from the Netherlands found that there was an increased probability of false positives due to rheumatoid factor with increasing age [34]. It has been recommended that sera should be routinely absorbed before MIF IgM testing. Some IgG antibody may result from a heterotypic response to other chlamydial species as there are cross-reactions with the MOMP between the three species as well as cross-reactions due to the genus LPS antigen. The omp1 gene which encodes for the MOMP is also highly conserved between the 4 chlamydial species with as much as 70 % conservation for nucleotide and amino acid sequences [7]. Moss and colleagues reported that antibodies to *C. pneumoniae* and *C. psittaci* accounted for up to half of all chlamydial IgG-positive persons attending a sexually transmitted disease clinic [27]. Cross-reactions have been described with other bacteria, specifically *Bartonella*, but cross-reactions with other species may also exist [25].

The MIF test is not standardized, there can be a significant subjective component in performing the assay. A recent study by Peeling et al. attempted to address the problem of interlaboratory variation in the performance of the MIF test by sending a panel of 22 acute and convalescent sera to 14 different laboratories in countries including the United States [29]. Some used an in-house MIF, several laboratories used one of two commercially available MIF kits (MRL and LabSystems). Both kits do not have FDA approval for this indication, the LabSystems kit is not available in the United States. The overall agreement of all laboratories was 80 %, using one laboratory as the "gold standard". The range was 50 % to 100 % depending on the isotype. Agreement for serodiagnostic criteria were 69 % for negative, 68 % for "chronic" and 87 % for a 4-fold increase of IgG.

Other serologic tests

The complement fixation (CF) test is widely available in many State laboratories. The test is genus specific using the chlamydial lipopolysaccharide antigen. It is used most frequently for the diagnosis of psittacosis and lymphogranuloma venereum. A four-fold titer rise or a titer $\geq 1:64$ with the CF test is also felt to be diagnostic for *C. pneumoniae* infection. Initially, it was found that fewer than one third of hospitalized patients with suspected *C. pneumoniae* infection had detectable CF antibody. In a report of a small outbreak of *C. pneumoniae* infections among University of Washington students, all seven patients with pneumonia had CF titers of 1:64 or greater [14]. However, in another study of community-acquired pneumonia in children, none of the children with culture-documented *C. pneumoniae* infection had CF antibody [13].

In an effort to circumvent the quality-control and subjective problems associated with the MIF assay, several serologic tests using ELISA-based formats have been developed. One, the rELISA Medac is commercially available in Europe [24]. It uses a recombinant, exclusively *Chlamydia* genus-specific fragment of the chlamydial LPS. The advantages of this test, suggested by the manufacturer, include the use of noninfectious and reproducible antigen, short performance time and objective reading. The test is genus specific and the diagnosis of infection is based on a rather complex combination of IgM, IgG and IgA results. Briefly of the 8 possible combinations, if IgG and IgA are positive this indicates acute infection; if the IgG is positive and the IgA is negative, this indicates past infection. If the IgG is negative and the IgA is positive, the manufacturer states that this may indicate the early stages of an active infection, and retesting in 10 to 14 days is indicated. These recommendations were not based on correlation with culture. Kutlin et al. compared this assay to the results of culture in adults and children with respiratory illness, including pneumonia and asthma [24]. The Medac assay with a single serum sample did not appear to be sensitive or specific for diagnosis of *C. pneumoniae* infection compared with the results of culture. In children, the sensitivity compared to culture was less than 35 %, with specificities < 91 %, depending on the isotype. In adults, the sensitivities were higher, up to 78 %, but the specificities ranged from a very low of 21 % for IgA or IgG to 81 % for IgM. When paired sera from culture-positive patients were tested, the results of the rELISA correlated with culture in 5 of 8 patients; 3 children remained seronegative by this assay. A recent study from Japan describes another ELISA which uses the *C. pneumoniae* major outer membrane complex as the antigen, theoretically, this should be more specific [28]. Although the authors found an "excellent correlation" between the results of the ELISA and MIF, 75 % and 64 % of 342 control children without respiratory symptoms had IgA and IgM antibodies to *C. pneumoniae* by MIF or ELISA. No comparison with culture or PCR was done.

An important confounding variable in the diagnosis of *C. pneumoniae* infection is the presence of asymptomatic infection. Results of several small studies have reported a rate of asymptomatic infection ranging from 2 % to 5 % in adults and children [4, 10, 12, 18]. These individuals were usually seronegative or had MIF IgG $\leq$ 1:256. There are no large, population-based studies that have examined the relationship of asymptomatic infection to age or serologic status. Persistent *C. pneumoniae* infection following acute respiratory infection has been reported and may last for several months to years. In following two patients who were persistently culture-positive for periods up to 9 years, their IgM and IgG titers fluctuated widely [9]. Combined with the observation that coinfections with other organisms, such as *Mycoplasma pneumoniae* and *Streptococcus pneumoniae*, are frequent in individuals with respiratory infection and positive *C. pneumoniae* cultures, it is possible that *C. pneumoniae* may be a cofactor or innocent bystander. Block et al. reported that 20 % of the children with culture-documented *C. pneumoniae* infection were coinfected with *M. pneumoniae*; these children could not be clinically differentiated from those who were infected with either agent alone [3].

Nonculture tests

Although PCR holds promise as a rapid diagnostic test, there are no standardized PCR or other nucleic acid amplification tests for detection of *C. pneumoniae*. The assays currently described in the literature are all in-house tests that employ different primers, the most frequently used have been those based on the omp1 gene, the 16S rRNA gene and a *C. pneumoniae*-specific DNA fragment [6, 11, 21, 31]. Some assays described are nested, and they appear to be more sensitive, but are more likely to be subject to contamination. These assays also use different methods for detection of the amplified gene product, including poly acrylamide gel electrophoresis, ethidium bromide staining and transillumination and hybridization with an RNA biotin-labeled probe followed by an enzyme immunoassay (EIAs). The PCR-EIA appears to be more sensitive than ethidium bromide stained gels [11]. However, none of these various PCR assays have been extensively evaluated compared to culture in respiratory specimens; thus their performance can vary greatly study-to-study. We compared a PCR-EIA using 16S rRNA-based primers to culture for detection of *C. pneumoniae* in NP specimens from 43 symptomatic and 58 asymptomatic individuals, PCR had a sensitivity compared to culture of 73 % and a specificity of 99 % [11]. In contrast, other investigators using the same primers in a hemi-nested assay found that PCR was significantly more sensitive than culture in throat swabs from children with respiratory illness, 15 of 368 (4 %) specimens were positive by PCR, but only one (0.2 %) was culture positive [21]. The difference in performance between these two studies could be due to the presence of DNA polymerase inhibitors in clinical specimens in the first study, making the PCR less sensitive. However, the improved performance of PCR in the second study could also be due to suboptimal culture methods. The prevalence of culture positivity was very low, only 0.2 %, which is 10-fold lower than the background rates of asymptomatic infection with *C. pneumoniae*, documented by culture, reported in several studies of children and adults.

The issue of comparability of PCR methods is especially important when one reviews the current literature on the relationship of *C. pneumoniae* and atherosclerosis. *C. pneumoniae* has been reported to be present by PCR in 0 to >90 % of samples of vascular tissue [36]. There has been one attempt to correlate the performance of PCR in various laboratories [32]. Samples of coronary arteries from 10 explanted hearts were sent to 9 different laboratories for culture, PCR, immunohistochemical staining and *in situ* hybridization. Two of the four laboratories that performed PCR used the 463-bp fragment of the 16S rRNA gene. The amplified gene product was detected by ethidium bromide staining of gels in one laboratory and by PCR-EIA in the other. The third laboratory used the *C. pneumoniae*-specific DNA fragment and the remaining laboratory used primers from the omp1 gene. One specimen was culture positive in all 3 laboratories that performed culture and was the only specimen positive by *in situ* hybridization. The specimen was also positive in 3 of the 4 laboratories that performed PCR. Of the remaining

9 culture-negative specimens, 4 were positive by PCR in only one of the 4 laboratories that performed PCR. There was also no correlation between MIF titers and evidence of *C. pneumoniae* by any method.

References

1. Augenbraun MH, Roblin PM, Mandel LJ, et al. (1991) *Chlamydia pneumoniae* pneumonia with pleural effusion: diagnosis by culture. Am J Med 91: 437–438
2. Black CM, Jonson JE, Farshy CE, et al. (1991) Antigenic variation among strains of *Chlamydia pneumoniae*. J Clin Microbiol 29: 1312–1316
3. Block S, Hedrick J, Hammerschlag MR, Cassell GH (1995) *Mycoplasma pneumoniae* and *Chlamydia pneumoniae* in community acquired pneumonia in children: Comparative safety and efficacy of clarithromycin and erythromycin suspensions. Pediatr Infect Dis J 14: 471–477
4. Block S, Hammerschlag MR, Hedrick J, et al. (1997) *Chlamydia pneumoniae* in acute otitis media. Pediatr Infect Dis J 16: 858–862
5. Campbell LA, Kuo CC, Wang SP, Grayston JT (1990) Serologic response to *Chlamydia pneumoniae* infection. J Clin Microbiol 28: 1261–1264
6. Campbell LA, Melgosa MP, Hamilton DJ, et al. (1992) Detection of *Chlamydia pneumoniae* by polymerase chain reaction. J Clin Microbiol 30: 434–439
7. Carter MW, Al-Mahdwawi SAH, Giles IG, et al. (1991) Nucleotide sequence and taxonomic value of the major outer membrane protein gene of *Chlamydia pneumoniae* IOL-207. J Gen Microbiol 137: 465–475
8. Cles L, Stamm WE (1990) Use of HL cells for improved isolation and passage of *Chlamydia pneumoniae*. J Clin Microbiol 28: 938–940
9. Dean D, Roblin P, Mandel L, et al. (1998) Molecular evaluation of serial isolates from patients with persistent *Chlamydia pneumoniae* infections. In: Stephens RS, Byrne GI, Christiansen G, Clarke IN, Grayston JT, Rank RG, Ridgway GL, Saikku P, Schachter J, Stamm WE (eds) Chlamydia infections. Proceedings of the Ninth International Symposium on Human Chlamydia Infections. University of California, San Francisco, pp. 219–222
10. Emre U, Roblin PM, Gelling M, et al. (1994) The association of *Chlamydia pneumoniae* infection and reactive airway disease in children. Arch Pediatr Adolesc Med 148: 727–731
11. Gaydos CA, Roblin PM, Hammerschlag MR, et al. (1994) Diagnostic utility of PCR-EIA, culture and serology for detection of *Chlamydia pneumoniae* in symptomatic and asymptomatic patients. J Clin Microbiol 32: 903–905
12. Gnarpe J, Gnarpe H, Sundelof B (1991) Endemic prevalence of *Chlamydia pneumoniae* in subjectively healthy persons. Scand J Infect Dis 23: 387–388
13. Grayston JT, Campbell L A, Kuo CC, et al. (1990) A new respiratory tract pathogen: *Chlamydia pneumoniae* strain TWAR. J Infect Dis 161: 618–625
14. Grayston JT, Aldous MB, Easton A, et al. (1993) Evidence that *Chlamydia pneumoniae* causes pneumonia and bronchitis. J Infect Dis 168: 1231–1235
15. Hammerschlag MR, Chirgwin K, Roblin PM, et al. (1992) Persistent infection with *Chlamydia pneumoniae* following acute respiratory illness. Clin Infect Dis 14: 178–182
16. Hammerschlag MR, Gregory W, Schwartz DB, et al. (1997) Azithromycin in the treatment of community-acquired pneumonia (CAP) due to *Chlamydia pneumoniae*. In Abstracts of

the 37th Interscience Conference on Antimicrobial Agents and Chemotherapy. American Society for Microbiology, Washington, DC. abstr. K-138, p. 352
17. Harris JA, Kolokathis A, Campbell M, et al. (1998) Safety and efficacy of azithromycin in the treatment of community acquired pneumonia in children. Pediatr Infect Dis J 17: 865–871
18. Hyman CL, Roblin PM, Gaydos CA, et al. (1995) The prevalence of asymptomatic nasopharyngeal carriage of *Chlamydia pneumoniae* in subjectively healthy adults: Assessment by polymerase chain reaction-enzyme immunoassay and culture. Clin Infect Dis 20: 1174–1178
19. Iijima Y, Miyashita N, Kishimoto T, et al. (1994) Characterization of *Chlamydia pneumoniae* species-specific protein immunodominant in humans. J Clin Microbiol 32: 583–588
20. Jantos CA, Heck S, Roggendorf R, et al. (1997) Antigenic and molecular analysis of different *Chlamydia pneumoniae* strains. J Clin Microbiol 35: 620–623
21. Jantos CA, Roggendorf R, Wuppermann FN, et al. (1998) Rapid detection of *Chlamydia pneumoniae* by PCR-enzyme immunoassay. J Clin Microbiol 36: 1890–1894
22. Kern DG, Neill MA, Schachter J (1993) A seroepidemiologic study of *Chlamydia pneumoniae* in Rhode Island. Chest 104: 208–213
23. Kutlin A, Roblin P, Hammerschlag MR (1998) Antibody response to *Chlamydia pneumoniae* infection in children with respiratory illness. J Infect Dis 177: 720–724
24. Kutlin A, Tsumura N, Roblin PM, Hammerschlag MR (1997) Evaluation of Chlamydia IgM, IgG, IgA rELISAs medac for diagnosis of *Chlamydia pneumoniae* infection. Clin Diag Lab Immunol 4: 213–216
25. Maurin M, Eb F, Etienne J, Raoult D (1997) Serological cross-reactions between *Bartonella* and *Chlamydia* species: implications for diagnosis. J Clin Microbiol 35: 2283–2287
26. Montalban GS, Roblin PM, Hammerschlag MR (1994) Performance of three commercially available monoclonal reagents for confirmation of *Chlamydia pneumoniae* in cell culture. J Clin Microbiol 32: 1406–1407
27. Moss TR, Darougar S, Woodland RM, et al. (1993) Antibodies to Chlamydia species in patients attending a genitourinary clinic and the impact of antibodies to *C. pneumoniae* and *C. psittaci* on the sensitivity and the specificity of *C. trachomatis* serology tests. Sex Transm Dis 20: 61–65
28. Numazaki K, Ikebe T, Chiba S (1996) Detection of serum antibodies against *Chlamydia pneumoniae* by ELISA. FEMS Immunol Med Microbiol 14: 179–183
29. Peeling RW, Wang SP, Grayston JT, et al. (1998) Chlamydia serology: Inter-laboratory variation in microimmunofluorescence results. In: Stephens RS, Byrne GI, Christiansen G, Clarke IN, Grayston JT, Rank RG, Ridgway GL, Saikku P, Schachter J, Stamm WE (eds) Chlamydia infections. Proceedings of the Ninth International Symposium on Human Chlamydia Infections. University of California, San Francisco, pp. 159–162
30. Peterson EM, Cheng X, Qu Z, de la Maza LM (1996) Characterization of the murine antibody response to peptides representing the variable domains of the major outer membrane protein of *Chlamydia pneumoniae*. Infect Immun 64: 3354–3359
31. Petitjean J, Vincent JPF, Fretigny M, et al. (1998) Comparison of two serological methods and a polymerase chain reaction-enzyme immunoassay for the diagnosis of acute respiratory infections with *Chlamydia pneumoniae* in adults. J Med Microbiol 47: 615–621

32. Ramirez JA, and the *Chlamydia pneumoniae*/Atherosclerosis Study Group (1996) Isolation of *Chlamydia pneumoniae* from the coronary artery of a patient with coronary atherosclerosis. Ann Intern Med 125: 979–982
33. Roblin PM, Dumornay W, Hammerschlag MR (1992) Use of HEp-2 cells for improved isolation and passage of *Chlamydia pneumoniae*. J Clin Microbiol 30: 1968–1971
34. Verkooyen RP, Hazenberg MA, Van Haaren GH, et al. (1992) Age-related interference with *Chlamydia pneumoniae* microimmunofluorescence serology due to circulating rheumatoid factor. J Clin Microbiol 30: 1287–1290
35. Wang SP, Grayston JT (1991) *Chlamydia pneumoniae* elementary body antigenic reactivity with fluorescent antibody is destroyed by methanol. J Clin Microbiol 29: 1539–1541
36. Weiss SM, Hammerschlag MR (1997) Are heart attacks infectious? A critical look at the link between *Chlamydia pneumoniae* and atherosclerosis. Bull Institut Pasteur 95: 107–113
37. Wong KH, Skelton SK, Chan YK (1992) Efficient culture of *Chlamydia pneumoniae* with cell lines derived from the human respiratory tract. J Clin Microbiol 30: 1625–1630

Discussion

Straube:

You have shown two or several patients with long-lasting Chlamydia infection with different results in the serology. Do you mean they have a chronic or a repeated infection?

Hammerschlag:

This is a very interesting point. We actually have several isolates of patients where the OMP1 have been sequenced by Debbie Dean at the UCSF, and they found what appeared to be transient minor changes in about two or three nucleotides, some of which were conformational. But they would often revert. It is hard to say. Intuitively I feel, because we have not seen this happen with other individuals, that the organisms are persisting. Obviously we might not be going after the right part of the genome that might be most important to look at. But based on some experience with children – some of whom have been infected for a long time – I think that this does represent the same organism and not reacquisition, otherwise these individuals have really bad luck.

Straube:

But the identical sequence does not answer this question because you can use the same source several times for infection.

Hammerschlag:

That is possible. Let us put it this way, we have followed patients whom we have treated and it goes away and does not appear to come back. It would be kind of difficult to hypothesize that these two individuals out of the hundreds that we followed have the bad luck of getting it 50 times, but we don't know. The other point is again there must be some way to differentiate between different strains, whether the organism is really all the same which is difficult to accept considering the wide geographic distribution.

Christiansen:

Maybe I can comment that. We analyzed about 10 different isolates coming from Finland, from ATCC, from Seattle by our long-range PCR and we found extremely rare changes. Of course we couldn't sequence it all, but in each case we selected a number of restriction enzymes that would cut frequently, looked for any kind of band variation in all those long-range PCR fragments and found only one region where 3 patients or 3 samples differed in the DNA-sequence.

Hammerschlag:

What is different geographically?

Christiansen:

MOMP seemed to be identical, momp-2 also seemed to be identical, the same was true for all the PMPs as well as omp-4-2.

Hammerschlag:

Where was the change?

Christiansen:

In some genes we do not know the function of.

Hammerschlag:

Maybe we get some more information as more strains become available to figure out what is going on. But I would like to point out again: we need a commercially available amplification test that is standardized, so that we all are doing the same thing. We need a good prospective study to work it out like it was done for *Chlamydia trachomatis*. When you think where we are with the diagnostic methods for *Chlamydia trachomatis* and where we are with *Chlamydia pneumoniae* – it is pathetic. In the United States we do not even have a commercially available species-specific culture confirmation reagent.

Byrne:

Maybe we could take a position on this as a result of this workshop, a comment on the status of the usefulness of serology. It would be useful if we could come to some consensus about that, whether we are talking about a test that actually does reflect an infection or a test that reflects exposure.

Chapter 3
Chronic Diseases Possibly Associated With *Chlamydia pneumoniae* Infections

3.1
Epidemiological data on respiratory tract infection with *Chlamydia pneumoniae* and clinical complications

J. Boman

A few epidemics of *Chlamydia pneumoniae* have been reported [1–4]. The first study linking *C. pneumoniae* to respiratory disease was performed by Saikku and colleagues in Finland and Seattle. Serum samples collected in 1978 from adolescents and young adults in two communities in northern Finland with chest X-ray infiltrates were investigated in Seattle by Saikku and Wang. The sera reacted in the microimmunofluorescence (MIF) test with a chlamydial strain – TW 183 – collected in Taiwan 1965. The study was published 1985 [1].

Grayston and colleagues performed a study of 386 university students with acute respiratory tract infection to determine whether *C. pneumoniae* is an important respiratory pathogen [5]. Serologic evidence of recent *C. pneumoniae* infection was found in 12 % of those with pneumonia, 5 % of those with bronchitis and 1 % of those with pharyngitis. Pharyngitis often accompanied by laryngitis was common in the early phase. The *C. pneumoniae* infections resembled clinically those with mycoplasma, causing mild pneumonias and prolonged illness. Prolonged illness or relapse of respiratory symptoms was commonly seen also in some students who got antibiotic therapy with macrolides.

Persistent carriage of *C. pneumoniae* following acute infection despite therapy with doxycycline or tetracycline was described by Hammerschlag and colleagues in 1992 [6]. They concluded that infection with *C. pneumoniae* may be very difficult to eradicate with use of currently available antibiotics even if there is a clinical response to therapy.

During 1993, 47 patients with acute or recent *C. pneumoniae* infection were diagnosed mainly by the MIF test at the Department of Clinical Virology, University Hospital of Northern Sweden, Umeå. Of these 47 patients, 38 were from the county of Västerbotten. During the first four months of 1994, an increase of 52 % in the *C. pneumoniae* incidence was observed, as compared to the same period in 1993. Out of 32 diagnosed cases of *C. pneumoniae* during the period, 14 (44 %) were from Byske, a village located in the northern part of Västerbotten. In 1994, there were 4,808 residents in Byske, representing 1.85 % of the population in Västerbotten. Most of the cases were pupils at the senior level of the nine-year compulsory school in Byske. As expected, several cases were also found among parents, siblings and teachers. The clinical picture among the patients with diagnosed *C. pneumoniae* infection included rhinitis, sore throat, hoarseness, fever, myalgia, protracted cough, arthralgia and fatigue [7].

As a result of this high accumulation of *C. pneumoniae* cases, we decided to perform a study for the evaluation of different diagnostic methods on different types of samples for early diagnosis of *C. pneumoniae* infection. Therefore, all patients during the period between May 1 and August 31, 1994 with a clinical suspicion of an acute *C. pneumoniae* infection who had consulted a physician at the Byske Primary Health Care Centre were offered to be included in the study. Eligible patients had respiratory symptoms and no other evident diagnosis. Attempts were made to collect a sputum sample, a nasopharyngeal swab, a throat swab, and paired serum samples from all patients. Respiratory samples were analyzed by means of nested touchdown PCR, culture in McCoy and HEp-2 cells, and *Chlamydia* genus-specific EIA. Serology was performed using the MIF and the CF tests.

From 129 persons, 319 respiratory samples and 153 serum samples were collected. By nested PCR, 30 patients were diagnosed with *C. pneumoniae* compared with 26 by EIA and 23 by culture. The finding of *C. pneumoniae* in the respiratory tract was accompanied by serology indicating acute infection in 26 of 27 patients from whom adequately collected serum samples were available. Sputum samples, when such samples could be obtained, were superior to throat and nasopharyngeal swabs. HEp-2 cells were more sensitive than McCoy cells, and positive EIA results needed confirmation by an alternative method. Serology by MIF was a useful complement to the detection methods to distinguish an acute infection from a carrier state.

Between January 1993 to September 1997 a total of 681 cases of respiratory chlamydial infection were diagnosed at the Department of Virology, University Hospital of Umeå. The majority – 436 cases (64 %) – occurred in 1995. With few exceptions, the respiratory chlamydial infections were caused by *C. pneumoniae*.

Most cases among boys/men occurred at the ages 9–22 and among girls/women at the ages 11–18 and 31–45. Few cases were diagnosed in young children aged 0–5 years (3/681; < 0.5 %). The number of patients treated for AMI, stroke or peri-myocarditis at Umeå University Hospital was recorded for a 7-year period: before, during and after the *C. pneumoniae* epidemic. When the epidemic occurred in the university town Umeå – spring 1995 – there were 100 or more diagnosed cases of peri-myocarditis compared to any of the other 13 six-month periods. This epidemiological link between *C. pneumoniae* and inflammatory heart disease is in line with a recently published study by Bachmaier et al. [8]. They showed that *Chlamydia* makes a peptide that mimics a portion of heart muscle protein. In mice, these peptides can trigger a severe inflammation of the heart. The number of cases with AMI was higher during and after the epidemic whereas the number of cases with stroke was similar before, during and after the *C. pneumoniae* epidemic.

References

1. Saikku P, Wang SP, Kleemola M, Brander E, Rusanen E, Grayston JT (1985) An epidemic of mild pneumonia due to an unusual strain of *Chlamydia psittaci*. J Infect Dis 15: 832–839
2. Grayston JT, Mordhorst C, Bruu AL, Vene S, Wang SP (1989) Countrywide epidemics of *Chlamydia pneumoniae*, strain TWAR, in Scandinavia, 1981-1983. J Infect Dis 159: 1111–1114
3. Ekman MR, Grayston JT, Visakorpi R, Kleemola M, Kuo CC, Saikku P (1993) An epidemic of infections due to *Chlamydia pneumoniae* in military conscripts. Clin Infect Dis 17: 420–425
4. Kleemola M, Saikku P, Visakorpi R, Wang SP, Grayston JT (1988) Epidemics of pneumonia caused by TWAR, a new *Chlamydia* organism, in military trainees in Finland. J Infect Dis 157: 230–236
5. Grayston JT, Kuo CC, Wang SP, Altman J (1986) A new *Chlamydia psittaci* strain, TWAR, isolated in acute respiratory tract infections. N Engl J Med 315(3): 161–168
6. Hammerschlag MR, Chirgwin K, Roblin PM, Gelling M, Dumornay W, Mandel L, Smith P, Schachter J (1992) Persistent infection with *Chlamydia pneumoniae* following acute respiratory illness. Clin Infect Dis 14: 178–182
7. Boman J, Allard A, Persson K, Lundborg M, Juto P, Wadell G (1997) Rapid diagnosis of respiratory *Chlamydia pneumoniae* infection by nested touchdown polymerase chain reaction compared with culture and antigen detection by EIA. J Infect Dis 175: 1523–1526
8. Bachmaier K, Neu N, de la Maza LM, Pal S, Hessel A, Penninger JM (1999) Chlamydia infections and heart disease linked through antigenic mimicry. Science 283: 1335–1339

Discussion

Anonymus:
Did you analyse the data on acute myocard infarction in people over 50 years old?

Boman:
Yes, and there was no difference compared to below the age of 50.

Byrne:
Are you continuing to follow this group? Because for infarction and stroke we may be talking about end stage for instance 5 or 10 years down the road, as opposed to myocarditis which seems to happen quickly.

Boman:
Yes, we know where the epidemic was located so we will follow the people living there. Within the Byske epidemic we compared different diagnostic methods. We followed all PCR-positive patients for two years. After two years they

were all PCR negative, and their serology (IgM) had reverted to negative in all of them. We have also sent out a questionnaire. Many of the patients reported persistent symptoms for several months following the acute infection which started during the epidemic and didn't disappear, for example asthma and arthralgia. However, we have not seen an increase in a coronary heart disease from this area. But we will continue to follow them.

Stille:

Maybe the first epidemic happened in Switzerland, describing Wassermann-positive pneumonia.

Anonymus:

In the 50s and 60s we had epidemics of ornithosis without contact with birds and they had the characteristic positive lues reactions, Wassermann's reaction, and so apparently these were the first epidemics I know of.

Boman:

Yes, I know about earlier descriptions of epidemics that probably were caused by *C. pneumoniae*. But the study by Saikku and colleagues was the first one specifically linking *C. pneumoniae* to disease in humans, since they had the TWAR antigen.

Hammerschlag:

The studies that we are involved in with *C. pneumoniae* are multicenter studies involving people from the States, every state and multiple centers. In the first one by Block complement fixation was done and none of the children were positive, even those who were culture-positive. Obviously if you are going to deal for instance with Brooklyn which has a population officially of 2.5 million, maybe unofficially 3.5, it is different from the point of view of socioeconomic factors compared to northern Sweden. We do not seem to have outbreaks per se but kind of a constant transmission in the city. It may explain some of the differences in serology because of the way it spreads through the population. Here we can get individual patients like what you have. It just does not seem to fit into this kind of very discrete an epidemic we have always. And it is not, for the most part, very severe, although we have had a few patients with empyema.

Boman:

It is the same in the southern part of Sweden, in Stockholm and in other big cities, where we don't identify *C. pneumoniae* epidemics. The reason may be that the northern part of Sweden is not a very crowded area. Similar patterns have been described in northern Finland, northern Sweden and northern Norway but not in the southern parts of these countries. Outbreaks have been reported with a frequency of about six years between the peaks. We did not see positives by CF test or MIF below the age of 5. So we are planning to collect samples of children in daycare centers during the next outbreak. Perhaps young children have such a mild disease that they don't seek medical care and we don't get samples from them.

Hammerschlag:

Except in our Block study, the children were between 3 and 12, and the Harris study went from 6 months to 16. In the children who are 3 to 5 and even the ones who were 6 months to about the same age, probable infection is defined at least by radiographic evidence of pneumonia. So they had to present with something. The other kids seemed to have much the same frequencies of infections as the older children.

Hense:

Just a critical comment: It is sometimes tempting when looking at disease rates – I am talking as an epidemiologist here – because it jumps at your eyes and it is first-sight diagnosis. But looking at it from a maybe more critical viewpoint, to me it was surprising to see that in the second half of '95 the rates *C. pneumoniae* infections dropped very low, they were about the lowest in the whole period that you were watching, although at the same time the outbreak reached its peak in the middle of '95. Is there any explanation of why all of a sudden you have such a collapse of disease rates of myocarditis? Were all the people that were susceptible sort of suffering of myocarditis? Or what happened there, because it dropped down drastically.

Boman:

The incidence of *C. pneumoniae* dropped when the school closed for the summer, therefore there was a dramatic decrease in disease. But we had cases during the fall for which I have no explanation. The only thing I know is that several of these cases with myocarditis were diagnosed with *C. pneumoniae*. I think that is a good start but we have to try to trace sera from these patients; sera collected before, during and after the epidemic. This is just an observation that is in agreement with the *Science* paper by Bachmaier et al. that *C. pneumoniae* may provoke an autoimmune disease.

Saikku:

Our experience with complement fixation is that in primary infections when the patients have IgM antibodies it is a very good test and IgM can be positive in first sample in 60 % of those patients. But when elderly patients get reinfection they are negative in complement fixation tests.

3.2
Role of *C. pneumoniae* in severe asthma and COPD: Epidemiology and treatment

R. Cosentini, F. Blasi

Asthma

Up to not long ago it was a common conception that bacterial infections play a minor role in asthma attacks [1]. Since the early 1990s the role of *Chlamydia pneumoniae* in exacerbations of asthma has been investigated. Hahn et al. [2] first reported a possible association between *Chlamydia pneumoniae* infection and adult-onset asthma. Later studies confirmed the etiological role of *Chlamydia pneumoniae* infection in both adult and children asthma exacerbations [3–6]. In adults *Chlamydia pneumoniae* is reported to cause approximately 10 % of asthma exacerbations [3,6]. Most studies described patients with mild to moderate exacerbations whereas a recent study by our group, while confirming the role of this pathogen in mild to moderate asthma exacerbations, suggests that *Chlamydia pneumoniae* must also be considered as a cause of severe asthma attacks [7] (Table 1).

Table 1. Demographic functional, serological and PCR data on patients with acute asthma exacerbations.

	Severe Asthma Exacerbations (PEF ≤ 50 % of predicted) (n=15)	Mild–Moderate Asthma Exacerbations (PEF > 50 % of predicted) (n=20)
Mean age	32.7 ± 9.9	32.2 ± 10.5
Males/Females	9/6	11/9
Mean FEV_1 on admission	0.58 ± 0.10 L/s	1.71 ± 0.33 L/s
Mean PEF on admission	147 ± 42.3 L/min	463 ± 85.2 L/min
Acute infection (serology)	9/15	2/20
C. pneumoniae PCR positivity on pharyngeal swab specimens in acute infection cases	6/9	1/2

FEV_1 = forced expiratory volume
PEF = peak expiratory flow

The role of *Chlamydia pneumoniae* infection in acute asthma exacerbations is further suggested by the fact that in asthma patients antibiotic treatment with clarithromycin reduces airway hyperresponsiveness [8].

The possible role of *C. pneumoniae* in chronic severe asthma has been further evaluated in a multinational study on the role of macrolide treatment in asthma.

We have examined the association between IgG and IgA titers to *C. pneumoniae* and the severity of asthma in the subjects who were screened for this study. In the screened population the use of high-dose inhaled steroids was associated with a 74 % increase in IgG antibody titers (p=0.035) and a 71 % increase in IgA antibody titers (p=0.0001) when compared with the use of low-dose inhaled steroids. We also observed an inverse association between IgG antibodies and FEV_1 (p=0.043). In this group IgA antibodies were also associated with higher daytime symptom score (p=0.036). This raises the possibility that chronic infection with *C. pneumoniae* leads to an increase in the severity of asthma.

Chronic bronchitis

The onset of chronic obstructive pulmonary disease (COPD) is primarily associated with cigarette smoking, although it is not clear whether the inflammatory changes found in the airways of smokers are sufficient to explain the severe limitations to airflow typical of the late stages of this disease [9]. Therefore, it has been suggested that other factors, including infections, may interact with cigarette smoking in the natural history of the disease [10]. Given that *Chlamydia trachomatis* infection is known to cause tissue derangement in chronic pelvic inflammatory disease, it may be supposed that chronic *Chlamydia pneumoniae* infection may promote similar tissue scarring mechanisms in the airways.

The association between *Chlamydia pneumoniae* infection and chronic bronchitis has been investigated and it appears that approximately 5 % of COPD acute exacerbations are sustained by this pathogen [11]. In the same study Blasi et al. found a significantly higher frequency of IgG anti-*Chlamydia pneumoniae* antibodies in patients with COPD exacerbations compared to controls [11]. It was suggested that this could be due either to chronic *Chlamydia pneumoniae* infection or to a higher rate of acute infections in these patients. Von Hertzen et al. [12] found no differences in serum IgG antibodies between patients and controls, whereas the difference in serum IgA prevalence was significant. Moreover, local sputum IgA antibodies against *Chlamydia pneumoniae*, absent in the majority of pneumonia patients, were a common finding in the sputa of chronic bronchitis patients, along with local antibodies towards bacteria more commonly associated with COPD such as *Haemophilus influenzae* and *Branhamella catarrhalis*.

A later study by von Hertzen et al. [13] on consecutive patients with COPD gave further proof of chronic *Chlamydia pneumoniae* infection in these patients given the stable IgA levels, the almost complete absence of seroconversions and the frequent presence of circulating immunocomplexes. In a later review [14], the same authors suggested that the elevated serum antibody levels and the presence of specific antibodies in sputum that are characteristic of *Chlamydia pneumoniae* involvement in COPD may indicate a biased Th2-type immune response with increased IL-4 and IL-10 production. IL-10 has been shown to induce IgA antibody production, and the high IgA levels found in COPD patients may reflect a defense mechanism to mitigate airway inflammation.

Although most of the above studies contained patients with mild-to-moderate COPD exacerbations, a recent study by Soler et al. investigated the etiological pattern of severe COPD exacerbations requiring mechanical ventilation [15]. Evidence of *Chlamydia pneumoniae* infection was found in 18 % of patients, although in almost a third of cases a mixed infection was present.

Table 2. Culture positivity in *C. pneumoniae* PCR-positive and -negative stable COPD patients.

PCR for *C. pneumoniae*	No. of Samples	No. of Bacteria	Total
Positive * (12 pts)	61	70	131
Negative (27 pts)	115	47	162
Total	176	117	293

* Chi-square test p<0.001

Whereas in healthy subjects the lower respiratory tract is usually sterile, in COPD patients bacterial colonization of the airways is common. In a recent study Blasi et al. (unpublished data) evaluated clinically stable COPD patients by obtaining at least 3 sputum samples from each patient at 4-week intervals. Quantitative culture was performed on sputum samples and a nested-PCR was applied for the detection of *Chlamydia pneumoniae* DNA (see Table 2). Sputum cultures in patients with *Chlamydia pneumoniae* infection yielded a significantly higher number of pathogens in comparison to *Chlamydia pneumonia*-negative patients. These data indicate that *Chlamydia pneumoniae* chronic infection may increase susceptibility to airway colonization by other pathogens.

In conclusion, *Chlamydia pneumoniae* infection seems to be associated with both the severity of chronic asthma and acute exacerbations of asthma. Similarly in COPD, infection with this microorganism may be a cause of mild, moderate or severe exacerbation and increase airway colonization by other pathogens.

References

1. Frick WE, Busse WW (1988) Respiratory infections: their role in airway responsiveness and pathogenesis of asthma. Clin Chest Med 9: 539–549
2. Hahn DL, Dodge RW, Golubjatnikov R (1991) Association of *Chlamydia pneumoniae* (strain TWAR) infection with wheezing, asthmatic bronchitis, and adult-onset asthma. JAMA 266: 225–230
3. Allegra L, Blasi F, Centanni S, et al. (1994) Acute exacerbations of asthma in adults: role of *Chlamydia pneumoniae* infection. Eur Respir J 7: 2165–2168
4. Emre U, Roblin PM, Gelling M, et al. (1994) The association of *Chlamydia pneumoniae* infection and reactive airway disease in children. Arch Pediatr Adolesc Med 148: 727–732
5. Cunningham AF, Johnston SL, Julious SA, et al. (1998) Chronic *Chlamydia pneumoniae* infection and asthma exacerbations in children. Eur Respir J 11: 345–349
6. Miyashita N, Kubota Y, Nakajiama M, et al. (1998) *Chlamydia pneumoniae* and exacerbations of asthma in adults. Ann Allergy Asthma Immunol 80: 405–409
7. Cosentini R, Gandino A, Tarsia P, et al. (submitted) Severe asthma exacerbations: role of acute *Chlamydia pneumoniae* infection. Eur Respir J

8. Allegra L, Blasi F, Cosentini R, et al. (1998) Treatment with clarithromycin in exacerbations of Asthma caused by *Chlamydia pneumoniae*. The fourth International Conference on the macrolides, azalides, streptogamins and ketolides, Barcelona, p.45
9. Lamb D (1995) Pathology. In: Calverly P, Pride N (eds) Chronic Obstructive Pulmonary Disease. London: Chapman and Hall, pp 9–34
10. Murphy TF, Sethi S (1992) Bacterial infection in chronic obstructive pulmonary disease. Am Rev Respir Dis 146: 1067–1083
11. Blasi F, Legnani D, Lombardo VM, et al. (1993) *Chlamydia pneumoniae* infection in acute exacerbations of COPD. Eur Respir J 6: 19–22
12. Von Hertzen L, Leinonen M, Koskinen R, et al. (1994) Evidence of persistence of *Chlamydia pneumoniae* infection in patients with COPD. In: Orfila J, Byrne GI, Cherneskey MA, et al. (eds) Chlamydial Infections. Bologna: Società Editrice Esculapio, pp 473–476
13. Von Hertzen L, Alakarppa H, Koskinen R, et al. (1997) *Chlamydia pneumoniae* infection in patients with chronic obstructive pulmonary disease. Epidemiol Infect 118: 155–164
14. Von Hertzen L (1998) *Chlamydia pneumoniae* and its role in chronic obstructive pulmonary disease. Ann Med 30: 27–37
15. Soler N, Torres A, Ewig S, et al. (1998) Bronchial microbial patterns in severe exacerbations of COPD requiring mechanical ventilation. Am J Respir Crit Care Med 157: 1498–1505

Discussion

Hammerschlag:

We found that most of the children with *C. pneumoniae* infection were not seropositive. We had one kid who was culture-positive on five occasions over a 6-month period before we finally made a riot about him taking his medication and he remained MIF-negative through the whole period. If the data are based on eradication of the organism, in our cases 75 % of the kids where we eradicated did improve somewhat dramatically, although we had some that did not, as demonstrated. Also we found that IgE antibody did not correlate at all with the MIF. Looking at adult patients with asthma and controls, our preliminary data show that the prevalence of infections defined by culture was the same as well as the antibody. Considering that macrolides and even tetracycline can have effects that are independent of their antimicrobial activity, I would think that in the roxithromycin study it would be very important to have a treatment group of patients who were seronegative because you are not treating the infection but something else. We have preliminary data working with our immunologist which were presented at the last immunology meetings. Looking at patients with severe asthma where we performed culture and serology, we found that almost everybody had antibodies as well as some of our controls. Minocyclin makes them better and also reduces the general levels of IgE which appears to be independent of the presence of any *C. pneumoniae* infection that we can define or find at that time.

Cosentini:

Thank you for your comment.

Byrne:
Are you talking about IgE in general or chlamydia-specific IgE?

Hammerschlag:
In the children we found chlamydia-specific IgE. But the reduction of IgE in the adult asthmatics is part of an ongoing study, but this is just general IgE.

Byrne:
That is kind of a surprise. Actually I think IgE is the one antibody that would be useful to look at, except for the comments that you made. I don't know that anyone has looked at that. It is difficult to measure IgE since most assays are not sensitive enough.

Hammerschlag:
We worked out an immunoassay that appears to be pretty good. But again we found an association in children which we don't find in adults. *Chlamydia pneumoniae* is an inflammatory trigger. There may be so many other inflammatory triggers going on in these patients, that it will be very hard to sort it out. The difference between the children and adults is very striking in our population.

Byrne:
I would like to comment about the COPD population in association with other pathogens. Are those any particular pathogens or general respiratory pathogens?

Cosentini:
Most of them were the pathogens that generally colonize the respiratory tract in COPD, *i.e.*: *S. pneumoniae, H. influenzae* and *M. catarrhalis*. But we also found gram-negative bacilli especially in the group with the most severe COPD state.

Stille:
Do you treat selected asthma patients with antibiotics and, if yes, which type of patients do you select? You have a 30-year-old physician and now he starts to get asthma. Will you treat him or will you not treat him?

Cosentini:
Not as a rule. I would treat him with macrolides if he were *Chlamydia pneumoniae* infected.

Stille:
If you discuss the item with doctors who are suffering from asthma, you will find several physicians who say, "oh, my asthma responds to antibiotics". And it is well known and has no explanation.

Cosentini:
That is an interesting comment.

3.3.1
Chlamydia pneumoniae in atherosclerosis

P. Saikku

Introduction

The previously proposed risk factors cannot explain the prevalence of coronary heart disease (CHD) and the most effective drugs against CHD, statins, do not prevent 70–80 % of the cases. New means to cure the leading cause of death all over the world are needed. The inflammatory nature of atherosclerosis underlying coronary heart disease is well established, and oxidized or enzymatically modified LDL have been the prime candidates as causes of this inflammation [1,2]. Recently, however, common viruses of the herpes virus group, dental infections, *H. pylori* infections and, first of all, infections caused by a common, obligatory intracellular, respiratory bacterial pathogen, *C. pneumoniae*, have been suggested to associate with CHD. Over the last years, several reviews [3–13] and numerous editorials on the subject appeared and seroepidemiological and histopathological findings were supported with results of animal experiments and preliminary intervention trials. In this review, principally the most recent findings are discussed; for earlier references, the reader is referred to the review by Mattila and others [9].

Epidemiological and seroepidemiological findings

The well-known phenomenon that acute infections can precipitate acute cardiovascular events [14] has been verified in a case-control analysis of 1,922 cases and 7,649 matched controls. An acute respiratory tract infection during two preceding weeks was a risk factor for AMI in persons without a history of clinical risk factors. The study, as also shown earlier [15], was unable to detect a special pathogen precipitating these events, but only the disease itself. Of the agents closely associated with CHD, only *C. pneumoniae* is common at the age of the maximum incidence of cardiovascular diseases, and a recent Italian study associated 12 of 61 serological reinfections by this agent with AMI in patients under 65 years of age [16]. The differentiation of reinfection from reactivation of a chronic infection was, however, not possible.

The association of *C. pneumoniae* with arteriosclerosis has now been verified in over twenty studies, and this trend continues [17–33]. Keeping in mind the publication bias of negative studies, there have so far been only a few negative studies [34–36]. The first used unmatched controls of different ethnic origin or hospital personnel occupationally exposed to *C. pneumoniae* infection. In the second study, the effect of an oncoming *C. pneumoniae* epidemic could not be excluded. Immunoblotting studies suggested that certain antigens could be more represented in *C. pneumoniae* immune response in CHD [28].

Histopathological studies

After the first electron microscopic demonstration of *C. pneumoniae* in atherosclerotic plaques by Shor et al. [37], there are now over twenty studies demonstrating the presence of *C. pneumoniae* in atherosclerotic lesions, and the agent is only rarely demonstrated in undamaged areas [38–60]. ICC, especially with antibody against a chlamydial group antigen, seems to be the most sensitive detection method, followed by nested PCR. Isolation of Chlamydia from lesions of chronic infections is difficult, but it has been successfully accomplished in atherosclerotic lesions [44, 48], and there is a recent report [54] describing an isolation percentage of 16 % when several passages were used, and this figure is comparable to that in trachoma, a chronic *C. trachomatis* infection, where the agent is much easier to culture than in *C. pneumoniae* infection. Besides coronary and carotid arteriosclerosis, *C. pneumoniae* has been detected also in abdominal aortic aneurysms [41, 42, 49, 56, 59] and aortic valves [50, 51, 55]. The prevalence of *C. pneumoniae* demonstrated by PCR from atherosclerotic lesions has varied from 0–2 % [34, 56] to 20–100 % [35–55, 57–60], possibly reflecting the difficulties in handling tissue samples with inhibitors and also the insensitivity of the PCR reaction when only one amplification round is used. Unfortunately, no standardized PCR method is available yet, and there seems to be a demand for standardized reagents, which could make the results mutually comparable.

Intervention trials

The first findings from preliminary intervention trials have already been published. The main interest in these trials was originally to study the effect of antibiotics on the markers of inflammation, but interesting data concerning *C. pneumoniae* were also obtained in two of these studies. Gupta et al. [61] chose from among 240 CHD cases 80 patients, with clearly elevated antibody titers against *C. pneumoniae*. Half of the patients received one or two courses of 1.5 g azithromycin and half only placebo. After 1.5 years, the rate of cardiac events in the placebo-treated patients with elevated antibody titers was 28 %, while in the treated group it was 8 % (p=0.025), which was similar to that in the group without antibodies. In the ROXIS study, Gurfinkel et al. [62] treated patients with unstable angina or non-q-wave myocardial infarction for one month daily with 150 mg of roxithromycin or with placebo. At 6 months the incidence of cardiac events was 1 vs. 9 in the groups of 93 treated and untreated patients, respectively (p=0.03). Effect was not persistent and in long-term statistical significance was lost [63]. In both studies, changes in inflammation markers were also seen. In a study on the effect of 4-month doxycycline treatment after by-pass surgery, not even the inflammation markers were affected [64]. Recently, in the ACADEMIC intervention study, an azithromycin course of three months did not effect on the rate of cardiac events nor antichlamydial antibodies, but inflammation markers were effected six months after the initiation of treatment [65]. All these studies have been preliminary and small-scale, and a critical editorial on antibiotic treatment at this moment has been published [66].

The incidence of and mortality from CHD has been in steady decline in developed countries since the 1960's. This has been explained to be due to alterations in dietary habits and risk factors, such as smoking and hypertension. Some authors point to the simultaneous advent of antibiotics effective against Chlamydia [67] and even propose the use of antibiotics to underlie the phenomenon called the "French paradox" [68]. Moreover, one should remember that antibiotics are also effective against *H. pylori* and dental infections. A recent study proposed a protective effect of tetracycline or fluoroquinolone courses from primary cardiac events [69]. The possible antimicrobial and anti-inflammatory effect of statins [70] which are currently used in the treatment of CHD should be kept in mind, too.

Possible pathogenetic mechanisms by which an infection could affect the development of atherosclerosis and coronary heart disease

There are several pathogenic mechanisms by which a pathogen could directly or indirectly induce atherogenesis, thrombosis and plaque rupture, which have been described in detail in the review by Danesh et al. [3]. The direct presence of the pathogen in plaques may induce a local inflammatory reaction associated with oxidative and proteolytic processes and with proliferative cell responses leading to lumen obstruction, thrombosis and plaque rupture. *C. pneumoniae* have been demonstrated in plaques, and several studies on the multiplication and induction of cytokine and adhesine production of *C. pneumoniae* have been published [71–77], as its predilection to cholesterol-filled smooth muscle cells [78]. Circulating immune complexes and chlamydial or *H. pylori* lipopolysaccharide (endotoxin of gram-negative bacteria) may damage the vascular endothelium. There are also several indirect effects by which a chronic inflammation can affect arteriosclerosis. Bacterial Hsp60 cross-reacts with its human counterpart and this has been suggested to lead to an autoimmunity process possibly playing a role in atherosclerosis [79]. Hsp60 is the antigen which has repeatedly been incriminated in chronic chlamydial infections [80]. Systemic infection leads to elevated levels of C-reactive protein, leukocyte count, and a variety of cytokines, all of them associated with arteriosclerosis. Even the classical risk factors, such as lowered HDL cholesterol, and elevated levels of fibrinogen and triglycerides and hypertension [81] can be found in chronic infections. An atherogenic lipid profile is associated with chronic *C. pneumoniae* infection in healthy males [82–84], possibly due to chronic induction of TNF. There is a possibility that the low risk factors connected with the metabolic syndrome are risk factors only in connection with a chronic *C. pneumoniae* infection [Leinonen, unpublished observation]. More direct evidence on the possible participation of *C. pneumoniae* in atherogenesis comes from the fact that macrophages infected with *C. pneumoniae* begin to uptake LDL cholesterol and transform to foam cells, the key cell in atherosclerosis [85]. The association of chronic *C. pneumoniae* infection with smoking and male gender [86, 87] demonstrated in several studies poses interesting questions. Is the susceptibility of males to chronic, iron-dependent *C. pneumoniae* infections [88] perhaps due to the higher iron load in men? To what extent are symptoms and signs associated with smoking due to its promoting effect on chronic *C. pneumoniae* infections, as demonstrated in a study on identical twins discordant for smoking [87]. Studies on the immunology of *C. pneumoniae* infection in CHD has but just started [89, 90].

All these processes could begin even in early childhood and manifest only at old age. Imbalance could develop gradually by deteriorating defense mechanisms, mostly due to age and accompanying diseases. Thus, for instance, an acute infection could activate a latent infection in the plaque and cause an AMI seen after episodes of acute infections, as described earlier.

Conclusions

The association of infections with CHD seems to be proven, but we do not know yet its importance for the disease process. We do not know what their significance as risk factors is, how we could find the patients possibly benefiting from anti-infection treatment, and what would then be proper treatment. The evidence seems to be most conclusive for *C. pneumoniae,* and several ongoing trials are to be completed at the turn of the century. If the results are positive and supported by *in vitro* and animal experiments, cardiology may be in for a revolution.

References

1. Ross R (1993) The pathogenesis of atherosclerosis: a perspective of the 1990s. Nature 362: 801–809
2. Bhakdi S, Dorweiler B, Kirchmann R (1995) On the pathogenesis of atherosclerosis enzymatic transformation of human low-density lipoprotein to an atherogenic moiety. J Exp Med 182: 1959–1971
3. Danesh J, Collins R, Peto R (1997) Chronic infections and coronary heart disease: is there a link? Lancet 350: 430–436
4. Ellis RW (1997) Infection and coronary heart disease. J Med Microbiol 46: 535–539
5. Gupta S, Camm AJ (1997) Chronic infection in the etiology of atherosclerosis – the case for *Chlamydia pneumoniae.* Clin Cardiol 20: 829–836
6. Libby P, Egan D, Skarlatos S (1997) Roles of infectious agents in atherosclerosis and restenosis. An assessment of the evidence and need for future research. Circulation 96: 4095–4103
7. Saikku P (1997) *Chlamydia pneumoniae* and atherosclerosis – an update. Scand J Infect Dis Suppl 104: 53–56
8. Coles KA, Plant AJ, Riley TV, Smith DW (1998) Cardiovascular disease – an infectious aetiology. Rev Med Microbiol 9: 17–27
9. Mattila KJ, Valtonen VV, Nieminen MS, Asikainen S (1998) Role of infection as a risk factor for atherosclerosis, myocardial infarction, and stroke. Clin Infect Dis 26: 719–734
10. Mehta JL, Saldeen TGP, Rand K (1998) Interactive role of infection, inflammation and traditional risk factors in atherosclerosis and coronary artery disease. J Am Coll Cardiol 31: 1217–1225
11. Muldowney JAS III (1998) *Chlamydia pneumoniae*: A treatable cause of atherosclerosis? Antimicr Infect Dis Newsletter 16: 1–4

12. Pai J, Knoop FC, Hunter WJ, Agrawal DK (1998) *C. pneumoniae* and occlusive vascular disease – identification and characterization. J Pharmacol Toxicol Methods 39: 51–61
13. Gupta S (1999) Chronic infection in the aetiology of atherosclerosis – focus on *Chlamydia pneumoniae*. Atherosclerosis 143: 1–6
14. Meier CR, Jick SS, Derby LE, Vasilakis C, Jick H (1998) Acute respiratory-tract infections and risk of first-time acute myocardial infarction. Lancet 351: 1467–1471
15. Mattila KJ (1989) Viral and bacterial infections in acute myocardial infarction. J Intern Med 225: 293–296
16. Blasi F, Cosentini R, Raccanelli R, Massari FM, Arosio C, Tarsia P, Allegra L (1997) A possible association of *Chlamydia pneumoniae* infection and acute myocardial infarction in patients younger than 65 years of age. Chest 112: 309–312
17. Saikku P, Leinonen M, Mattila K, Ekman MR, Nieminen MS, Mäkelä PH, Huttunen J, Valtonen V (1988) Serologic evidence of an association of a novel Chlamydia, TWAR, with chronic coronary heart disease and acute myocardial infarction. Lancet ii: 983–985
18. Leinonen M, Linnanmäki E, Mattila K, Nieminen MS, Valtonen V, Leirisalo-Repo M, Saikku P (1990) Circulating immune complexes containing Chlamydial lipopolysaccharide in acute myocardial infarction. Microb Pathog 9: 67–73
19. Thom DH, Wang SP, Grayston JT, Siscovick DS, Stewart DK, Kronmal RA, Weiss NS (1991) *Chlamydia pneumoniae* strain TWAR antibody and angiographically demonstrated coronary artery disease. Arterioscler Thromb 11: 547–551
20. Thom DH, Grayston JT, Siscovick DS, Wang SP, Weiss NS, Daling JR (1992) Association of prior infection with *Chlamydia pneumoniae* and angiographically demonstrated coronary artery disease. JAMA 268: 68–72
21. Melnick SL, Shahar E, Folsom AR, Grayston JT, Sorlie PD, Wang SP, Szklo M (1993) Past infection by *Chlamydia pneumoniae* strain TWAR and asymptomatic carotid atherosclerosis. Am J Med 95: 499–504
22. Linnanmäki E, Leinonen M, Mattila K, Ekman MR, Nieminen MS, Valtonen V, Saikku P (1993) Presence of *Chlamydia pneumoniae* specific antibodies in circulating immune complexes in coronary heart disease. Circulation 87: 1130–1134
23. Mendall MA, Carrington D, Strachan D, Patel P, Molineaux N, Levi J, Toosey T, Camm AJ, Northfield TC (1995) *Chlamydia pneumoniae*: Risk factors for seropositivity and association with coronary heart disease. J Infect 30: 121–128
24. Miettinen H, Lehto S, Saikku P, Haffner SM, Rönnemaa T, Pyörälä K, Laakso M (1996) Association of *Chlamydia pneumoniae* and acute coronary heart disease events in non-insulin-dependent diabetic and non-diabetic subjects in Finland. Eur Heart J 17: 682–688
25. Ossewaarde JM, Feskens EJM, De Vries A, Vallinga CE, Kromhout D (1998) *Chlamydia pneumoniae* is a risk factor for coronary heart disease in symptom-free elderly men, but *Helicobacter pylori* and cytomegalovirus are not. Epidemiol Infect 120: 93–99
26. Diedrichs H, Schneider CA, Scharkus S, Pfister H, Erdmann E (1997) Prevalence of chlamydial antibodies in patients with CHD [In German]. Herz Kreisl 29: 304–307
27. Lindberg G, Råstam L, Lundblad A, Sorlie PD, Folsom AR, ARIC Study Investigators (1997) The association between serum sialic acid and asymptomatic carotid atherosclerosis is not related to antibodies to Herpes type viruses or *Chlamydia pneumoniae*. Int J Epidemiol 26: 1386–1391

28. Maass M, Gieffers J (1997) Cardiovascular disease risk from prior *Chlamydia pneumoniae* infection can be related to certain antigens recognized in the immunoblot profile. J Infect 35: 171–176
29. Thomas GN, Scheel O, Koehler AP, Bassett DCJ, Cheng AFB (1997) Respiratory chlamydial infections in a Hong Kong teaching hospital and association with coronary heart disease. Scand J Infect Dis Suppl 104: 30–33
30. Cook PJ, Honeybourne D, Lip GYH, Beevers DG, Wise R, Davies P (1998) *Chlamydia pneumoniae* antibody titers are significantly associated with acute stroke and transient cerebral ischemia – the West Birmingham stroke project. Stroke 29: 404–410
31. Mazzoli S, Tofani N, Fantini A, Semplici F, Bandini F, Salvi A, Vergassola R (1998) *Chlamydia pneumoniae* antibody response in patients with acute myocardial infarction and their follow-up. Am Heart J 135: 15–20
32. Strachan DP, Carrington D, Mendall MA, Ballam L, Morris J, Butland BK, Sweetnam PM, Elwood PC (1999) Relation of *Chlamydia pneumoniae* serology to mortality and incidence of ischaemic heart disease over 13 years in the Caerphilly prospective heart disease study. Br Med J 318: 1035–1039
33. Fagerberg B, Gnarpe J, Gnarpe H, Agewall S, Wikstrand J (1999) *Chlamydia pneumoniae* but not cytomegalovirus antibodies are associated with future risk of stroke and cardiovascular disease – A prospective study in middle-aged to elderly men with treated hypertension. Stroke 30: 299–305
34. Weiss SM, Roblin PM, Gaydos CA, Cummings P, Patton DL, Schulhoff N, Shani E, Frankel R, Penney K, Quinn TC, Hammerschlag MR, Schachter J (1996) Failure to detect *Chlamydia pneumoniae* in coronary atheromas of patients undergoing atherectomy. J Infect Dis 173: 957–962
35. Kark J, Leinonen M, Paltiel O, Saikku P (1997) *Chlamydia pneumoniae* and acute myocardial infarction in Jerusalem. Int J Epidemiol 26: 730–738
36. Ridker PM, Kundsin RB, Stampfer J, Poulin S, Hennekens CH (1999) Prospective study of *Chlamydia pneumoniae* IgG seropositivity and risks of future myocardial infarction. Circulation 99: 1161–1164
37. Shor A, Kuo CC, Patton DL (1992) Detection of *Chlamydia pneumoniae* in coronary arterial fatty streaks and atheromatous plaques. S Afr Med J 82: 158–160
38. Kuo CC, Gown AM, Benditt EP, Grayston JT (1993) Detection of *Chlamydia pneumoniae* in aortic lesions of atherosclerosis by immunocytochemical stain. Arterioscler Thromb 13:1501–1504
39. Kuo CC, Grayston JT, Campbell LA, Goo YA, Wissler RW, Benditt EP (1995) *Chlamydia pneumoniae* (TWAR) in coronary arteries of young adults (15–34 years old). Proc Natl Acad Sci USA 92: 6911–6914
40. Campbell LA, O'Brien ER, Cappuccio AL, Kuo CC, Wang SP, Stewart D, Patton DL, Cummings PK, Grayston JT (1995) Detection of *Chlamydia pneumoniae* TWAR in human coronary atherectomy tissues. J Infect Dis 172: 585–588
41. Blasi F, Denti F, Erba M, Cosentini R, Raccanelli R, Rinaldi A, Fagetti L, Esposito G, Ruberti U, Allegra L (1996) Detection of *Chlamydia pneumoniae* but not *Helicobacter pylori* in atherosclerotic plaques of aortic aneurysms. J Clin Microbiol 34: 2766–2769
42. Ong G, Thomas BJ, Mansfield AO, Davidson BR, Taylor-Robinson D (1996) Detection and widespread distribution of *Chlamydia pneumoniae* in the vascular system and its possible implications. J Clin Pathol 49: 102–106

43. Muhlestein JB, Hammond EH, Carlquist JF, Radicke E, Thomson MJ, Karagounis LA, Woods ML, Anderson JL (1996) Increased incidence of Chlamydia species within the coronary arteries of patients with symptomatic atherosclerotic versus other forms of cardiovascular disease. J Am Coll Cardiol 27: 1555–1561
44. Ramirez JA, *Chlamydia pneumoniae*/atherosclerosis Study Group (1996) Isolation of *Chlamydia pneumoniae* from the coronary artery of a patient with coronary atherosclerosis. Ann Intern Med 125: 979–982
45. Chiu B, Viira E, Tucker W, Fong IW (1997) *Chlamydia pneumoniae*, cytomegalovirus, and herpes complex virus in atherosclerosis of the carotid artery. Circulation 96: 2144–2148
46. Kuo CC, Coulson AS, Campbell LA, Capuccio AL, Lawrence RD, Wang SP, Grayston JT (1997) Detection of *Chlamydia pneumoniae* in atherosclerotic plaques in the walls of arteries of lower extremities from patients undergoing bypass operation for arterial obstruction. J Vascul Surg 26: 29–31
47. Jackson LA, Campbell LA, Schmidt RA, Kuo CC, Capuccio AL, Lee MJ, Grayston JT (1997) Specificity of detection of *Chlamydia pneumoniae* in cardiovascular atheroma – evaluation of the innocent bystander hypothesis. Am J Pathol 150: 1785–1790
48. Jackson LA, Campbell LA, Kuo CC, Rodriguez DI, Lee A, Grayston JT (1997) Isolation of *Chlamydia pneumoniae* from a carotid endarterectomy specimen. J Infect Dis 176: 292–295
49. Juvonen J, Laurila A, Alakärppä H, Leinonen M, Surcel HM, Juvonen T, Kairaluoma M, Saikku P (1997) Demonstration of *Chlamydia pneumoniae* in the walls of abdominal aortic aneurysms. J Vascul Surg 25: 499–505
50. Juvonen J, Laurila A, Juvonen T, Alakärppä H, Surcel HM, Lounatmaa K, Kuusisto J, Saikku P (1997) Detection of *Chlamydia pneumoniae* in human non-rheumatic stenotic aortic valves. J Am Coll Cardiol 29: 1054–1059
51. Juvonen J, Juvonen T, Laurila A, Kuusisto J, Bodian CA, Alarakkola E, Särkioja T, Kairaluoma MI, Saikku P (1998) Can degenerative tricuspid aortic valve stenosis be caused by a persistent *Chlamydia pneumoniae* infection? Ann Int Med 128: 741–744
52. Kuo CC, Coulson AS, Campbell LA, Capuccio AL, Lawrence RD, Wang SP, Grayston JT (1997) Detection of *Chlamydia pneumoniae* in atherosclerotic plaques in the walls of arteries of lower extremities from patients undergoing bypass operation for arterial obstruction. J Vascul Surg 26: 29–31
53. Maass M, Krause E, Engel PM, Kruger S (1997) Endovascular presence of *C. pneumoniae* in patients with hemodynamically effective carotid artery stenosis. Angiology 48: 699–706
54. Maass M, Bartels C, Engel PM, Mamat U, Sievers HH (1998) Endovascular presence of viable *Chlamydia pneumoniae* is a common phenomenon in coronary artery disease. J Am Coll Cardiol 31: 827–832
55. Nyström-Rosander C, Thelin S, Hjelm E, Lindquist O, Påhlson C, Friman G (1997) High incidence of *Chlamydia pneumoniae* in sclerotic heart valves of patients undergoing aortic valve replacement. Scand J Infect Dis 29: 361–365
56. Petersen E, Boman J, Persson K, Arnerlov C, Wadell G, Juto P, Eriksson A, Dahlen G, Angquist KA (1998) *Chlamydia pneumoniae* in human abdominal aortic aneurysms. Eur J Vasc Endovasc Surg 15: 138–142
57. Taylor-Robinson D, Ong G, Thomas BJ, Rose ML, Yacoub MH (1998) *Chlamydia pneumoniae* in vascular tissue from heart transplant donors. Lancet 351: 1255
58. Yamashita K, Ouchi K, Shirai M, Gondo T, Nakazawa T, Ito H (1998) Distribution of *Chlamydia pneumoniae* infection in the atherosclerotic carotid artery. Stroke 29: 773–778

59. Lindholt JS, Ostergard L, Henneberg EW, Fasting H, Andersen P (1998) Failure to demonstrate *Chlamydia pneumoniae* in symptomatic abdominal aortic aneurysms by a nested polymerase chain reaction. Eur J Vasc Endovasc Surg 15: 161–164
60. Bartels C, Maass M, Bein G, Malisius R, Brill N, Bechtel JFM, Sayk F, Feller AC, Sievers HH (1999) Detection of *Chlamydia pneumoniae* but not cytomegalovirus in occluded saphenous vein coronary artery bypass grafts. Circulation 99: 879–882
61. Gupta S, Leatham EW, Carrington D, Mendall MA, Kaski JC, Camm AJ (1997) Elevated *Chlamydia pneumoniae* antibodies, cardiovascular events, and azithromycin in male survivors of myocardial infarction. Circulation 96: 404–407
62. Gurfinkel E, Bozovich G, Daroca A, Beck E, Mautner B, Roxis Study Group (1997) Randomised trial of roxithromycin in non-Q-wave coronary syndromes: ROXIS pilot study. Lancet 350: 404–407
63. Gurfinkel E, Bozovich G, Beck E, Testa E, Livellara B, Mautner B (1999) Treatment with the antibiotic roxithromycin in patients with acute non-Q-wave coronary syndromes – The final report of the ROXIS study. Eur Heart J 20: 121–127
64. Sinisalo J, Mattila K, Nieminen MS, Valtonen V, Syrjälä M, Sundberg S, Saikku P (1998) The effect of prolonged doxycycline therapy on *Chlamydia pneumoniae* serological markers, coronary heart disease risk factors and forearm basal nitric oxide production. J Antimicrob Chemother 41: 85–92
65. Anderson JL, Muhlestein JB, Carlquist J, Allen A, Trehan S, Nielson C, Hall S, Brady J, Egger M, Horne B, Lim T (1999) Randomized secondary prevention trial of azithromycin in patients with coronary artery disease and serologic evidence for *Chlamydia pneumoniae* infection. The azithromycin in coronary artery disease: elimination of myocardial infection with chlamydia (ACADEMIC) study. Circulation 99: 1540–1547
66. Grayston JT (1998) Antibiotic treatment of *Chlamydia pneumoniae* for secondary prevention of cardiovascular events. Circulation 97: 1669–1670
67. Ånestad G, Scheel O, Hungnes O, Marchioli R, di Pasquale A, Marfisis RM, Tognoni G, GISSI investigators, Gurfinkel E, Mautner B, Vaughan CJ, Hallwell B, Constans J, Seigner M, Blann A, Corri C (1997) Chronic infections and coronary heart disease (correspondence). Lancet 350: 1028–1030
68. Stille W, Dittmann R, Justnubling G (1997) Atherosclerosis due to chronic arteritis caused by *Chlamydia pneumoniae* – a tentative hypothesis. Infection 25: 281–285
69. Meier CR, Derby LE, Jick SS, Vasilakis C, Jick H (1999) Antibiotics and risk of subsequent first-time acute myocardial infarction. JAMA 281: 427–431
70. Vaughan CJ, Murphy MB, Buckley BM (1996) Statins do more than just lower cholesterol. Lancet 348: 1079–1082
71. Fryer RH, Schwobe EP, Woods ML, Rodgers GM (1997) Chlamydia species infect human vascular endothelial cells and induce procoagulant activity. J Investig Med 45: 168–174
72. Gaydos CA, Summersgill JT, Sahney NN, Ramirez JA, Quinn TC (1996) Replication of *Chlamydia pneumoniae* in vitro in human macrophages, endothelial cells, and aortic artery smooth muscle cells. Infect Immun 64: 1614–1620
73. Godzik KL, O'Brien ER, Wang SK, Kuo CC (1995) *In vitro* susceptibility of human vascular wall cells to infection with *Chlamydia pneumoniae*. J Clin Microbiol 33: 2411–2414
74. Heinemann M, Susa M, Simnacher U, Marre R, Essig A (1996) Growth of *Chlamydia pneumoniae* induces cytokine production and expression of CD14 in a human monocytic cell line. Infect Immun 64: 4872–4875

75. Kaukoranta-Tolvanen SS, Ronni T, Leinonen M, Saikku P, Laitinen K (1996) Expression of adhesion molecules on endothelial cells stimulated by *Chlamydia pneumoniae*. Microb Pathog 21: 407–411
76. Kaukoranta-Tolvanen SS, Teppo AM, Laitinen K, Saikku P, Linnavuori K, Leinonen M (1996) Growth of *Chlamydia pneumoniae* in cultured human peripheral blood mononuclear cells and induction of a cytokine response. Microb Pathog 21: 215–221
77. Molestina RE, Dean D, Miller RD, Ramirez JA, Summersgill JT (1998) Characterization of a strain of *Chlamydia pneumoniae* isolated from a coronary atheroma by analysis of the omp1 gene and biological activity in human endothelial cells. Infect Immun 66: 1370–1376
78. Knoebel E, Vijayagopal P, Figueroa JE II, Martin DH (1997) *In vitro* infection of smooth muscle cells by *Chlamydia pneumoniae*. Infect Immun 65: 503–506
79. Xu Q, Willeit J, Marosi M, Kleindienst R, Oberhollenzer F, Kiechl S, Stulning T, Luef G, Wick G (1993) Association of serum antibodies to heat-shock protein 65 with carotid atherosclerosis. Lancet 341: 255–259
80. Ward ME (1995) The immunobiology and immunopathology of chlamydial infection. APMIS 103: 769–796
81. Cook PJ, Lip GYH, Davies P, Beevers DG, Wise R, Honeyborne D (1998) *Chlamydia pneumoniae* antibodies in severe essential hypertension. Hypertension 31: 589–594
82. Laurila AL, Bloigu A, Näyhä S, Hassi J, Leinonen M, Saikku P (1997) *Chlamydia pneumoniae* antibodies and serum lipids in Finnish men: cross-sectional study. Br Med J 314: 1456–1457
83. Laurila A, Bloigu A, Näyhä S, Hassi J, Leinonen M, Saikku P (1997) Chronic *Chlamydia pneumoniae* infection is associated with a serum lipid profile known to be a risk factor for atherosclerosis. Arterioscler Thromb Vasc Biol 17: 2910–2913
84. Murray LJ, O'Reilly DPJ, Ong GML, O'Neill C, Evans AE, Bamford KB (1999) *Chlamydia pneumoniae* antibodies are associated with an atherogenic lipid profile. Heart 81: 239–244
85. Kalayoglu MV, Byrne GI (1998) Induction of macrophage foam cell formation by *Chlamydia pneumoniae*. J Infect Dis 177: 725–729
86. Karvonen M, Tuomilehto J, Pitkäniemi J, Naukkarinen A, Saikku P (1994) Importance of smoking for *Chlamydia pneumoniae* seropositivity. Int J Epidemiol 23: 1315–1321
87. Hertzen L von, Surcel HM, Kaprio J, Koskenvuo M, Bloigu A, Leinonen M, Saikku P (1998) Immune responses to *Chlamydia pneumoniae* in twins in relation to gender and smoking. J Med Microbiol 47(5): 441–446
88. Freidank HM, Billing H (1997) Influence of iron restriction on the growth of *Chlamydia pneumoniae* TWAR and *Chlamydia trachomatis*. J Clin Microbiol Infect 3(Suppl 2): 193
89. Halme S, Syrjälä H, Bloigu A, Saikku P, Leinonen M, Airaksinen J, Surcel HM (1997) Lymphocyte responses to chlamydia antigens in patients with coronary heart disease. Eur Heart J 18: 1095–1101
90. Mosorin M, Surcel HM, Laurila A, Saikku P, Juvonen T (1998) *Chlamydia pneumoniae* reactive T lymphocytes in atherosclerotic plaque of carotid artery. In: Stephens RS, Byrne GI, Christiansen G, Clarke IN, Grayston JT, Rank RG, Ridgway GL, Saikku P, Schachter J, Stamm WE (eds) Chlamydia infections. Proceedings of the Ninth International Symposium on Human Chlamydia Infections. University of California, San Francisco, pp 423–425

Discussion

Bhakdi:

We have been discussing two possible contributions of infection towards atherosclerosis. The first would be that the infection is the cause and the second that the infection can drive atherogenesis and cause exacerbation. The last scheme that you showed is taking us a very long way back in saying that the infection is the cause. Would you yourself have any problems with the fact that many people fail to find *C. pneumoniae* in plaques, even in the older plaques? Because if we are looking at this as a risk factor for progression then we can say, it is all right if 10 or 20 % have them in the plaques. But if you say it is the cause, don't you think we should see this in very early lesions? I do not believe that there are any documented good data showing the presence of *C. pneumoniae* in early lesions.

Saikku:

Dr. Taylor Robinson has found *C. pneumoniae* already in boys 14 years of age in early lesions so that it seems to sit in the vessel wall quite early. And Dr. Shore who first found *C. pneumoniae* in atherosclerotic plaques realized that those curious round structures are *C. pneumoniae* particles. He is convinced that if you go through the atherosclerotic plaques very thoroughly, you will find it in 100 %. Of course there is a possibility of a hit-and-run occasion, then it would be very difficult to find. But we have heard today that PCR has problems, immunohistochemistry has problems and the isolation has problems, so at the moment I think some 80 % atherosclerotic plaques can be positive with the *C. pneumoniae*. But I cannot say that Dr. Shore is wrong.

Maass:

We will have time later for the pro and contra discussion, and I think it is a very basic problem to decide which methods are sensitive, which are specific and which are reliable. I think it is a very important contribution.

Hense:

If I understood your last slide correctly, it seemed to implicate that you have the plaques first and, as a consequence of a chronic persistent infection in plaques, you get increase of blood pressure, you get raised blood lipid levels. Would you try to explain to me because so far my understanding was the other way round.

Saikku:

I think these are different types of manifestation, they are typical for chronic inflammation and continuous induction of cytokines. And it is well-known that these cytokines effect very many different symptoms, like for instance fatigue and tiredness. One could speculate that these elevated cytokine levels then could lead to many alterations in the individual which are counted as risk factors, although they are only reflections of the continuous process. For instance, movement-reduced physical activity can be due to chronic inflammation which produces cytokines and leads to fatigue. Of course, if you exercise them, then it peps up their immune defense system, too.

Hense:

How do you then explain that you reduce the risk when lowering lipids and lowering blood pressure?

Saikku:

Statins are effective only in those persons who have a chronic inflammation, and this can, at least partly, be due to their antiinflammatory effect. They are also effective in normal cholesterinemic persons without lipid disturbances. We have not studied those blood pressure-lowering drugs which are effecting on calcium channels. Calcium channels are very important in chlamydial infections.

3.3.2
Prevalence of *Chlamydia pneumoniae* in human coronary plaques with acute coronary syndrome

G. Bauriedel, U. Welsch and B. Lüderitz

Introduction

A body of data have suggested that atherosclerosis is primarily an inflammatory disease [1–5]. In this context, the infectious hypothesis is attracting growing attention [5–10]. Various microorganisms have been discussed as the causative pathogen, such as cytomegalo-, herpes and influenza viruses, *Mycoplasma pneumoniae*, streptococci, staphylococci, *Helicobacter pylori*, but especially *Chlamydia pneumoniae* [5–13].

Table 1. Prevalence of *C. pneumoniae* in different cardiovascular diseases/tissues from patients.

Tissue	N	IHC positive	PCR positive	IHC/PCR positive	Authors
Aortic aneurysms	51		50 %		Blasi et al. [27]
Carotid plaques	76	71 %			Chiu et al. [28]
Aortic valve degeneration	27			63 %	Juvonen et al. [29]
Coronary atherectomy samples	90	79 %			Muhlestein et al. [12]
Coronary atherectomy samples	38	45 %	32 %	55 %	Campbell et al. [13]
Coronary autopsy tissue (age 15–34 yrs.)					Kuo et al. [30]
High grade lesions	7	86 %			
Intimal hyperplasia	11	18 %			
Intact artery/ mammarial artery	31	0 %			

ICH = immunohistochemistry
PCR = polymerase chain reaction

Considerations of the role of *C. pneumoniae* in human atherosclerosis have predominantly been based on various seroepidemiologic and histopathologic findings [5–10,12–14]. There are several cardiovascular settings in which the presence of this microorganism has been shown (Table 1). However, as to atherosclerosis, the specific *C. pneumoniae*-transmitted processes that act on the intimal microecology of the vascular wall are still uncertain. From the clinical perspective, questions arise for a prevalence of *C. pneumoniae* with certain types of human atherosclerosis. Possibly, there is a prevalence of the microorganism with atheroma types that predispose to or are even implicated in plaque rupture. Therefore, the present study was aimed to demonstrate *C. pneumoniae* in human coronary atherectomy samples from symptomatic patients, to compare the intralesional findings obtained from acute coronary syndrome and stable atheroma, and to assess for a relationship with characteristic structural features of the lesions.

Patients and methods

Patients and Plaque Tissue. Coronary plaque tissue of primary lesions from 51 patients was retrospectively examined after directional atherectomy [15] for the presence of *C. pneumoniae* by use of immunohistochemistry and transmission electron microscopy. The diagnosis "acute coronary syndrome" was based on a detailed patient history as well as individual clinical findings, and was categorized according to the criteria of Braunwald [16]. The intralesional findings associated with clinically acute coronary syndrome according to Braunwald's classification (n=31) were compared to those with stable angina (n=20) and regarded for potential relations to characteristic plaque features.

Immunohistochemistry. Removed plaque tissue was fixed in 4 % buffered formaldehyde and embedded in paraffin. Semi-thin sections (4 µm) were prepared from these segments for immunohistochemical investigation. The tissue was analyzed qualitatively for the incidence of specific structural features as well as for demonstrating the microorganism. The presence of *C. pneumoniae* was detected by immunohistochemical identification of the *C. pneumoniae*-specific epitome on the surface protein OMP1 of inclusion bodies by means of monoclonal antibodies (Medac Inc., Hamburg). Methodical details of the pretreatment steps, subsequent staining procedure (APAAP, Fast Red), and morphometric assessment followed the instructions of the manufacturer and recent reports [17, 18]. *C. pneumoniae*-infected epithelial mammalian cells (Medac Inc., Hamburg) served as positive controls.

Transmission Electron Microscopy (TEM). After atherectomy, tissue samples were fixed in 3.5 % glutaraldehyde; further steps of the methods applied have been recently described [17–20]. TEM proved to be especially useful for the specific detection of chlamydial structures, i.e. cytoplasmic reticular bodies or intra- and extracellular elementary bodies. The analysis was based on specific morphologic features, as recently published [11–13, 21].

Statistical Analysis. Probability calculations were done by the Mann-Whitney U test, all calculated probability values corrected by random sampling. Values of $p<0.05$ were considered to be statistically significant. The data were expressed as mean values ± standard deviation (SD).

Results

Immunoreaction for *C. pneumoniae* was found in 32 of 51 (63 %) coronary plaques. Signals were present with necrotic areas (40 %), sparse cellularity (40 %), neo-vascularization (29 %), thrombi (20 %), ruptured plaque areas (19 %), and fields rich in foam cells and calcifications. Intimal hyperplasia and inflammatory infiltrates showed no signals. As the central finding in this report, *C. pneumoniae* immunoreaction was more frequently ($p<0.001$) found in 26 of 31 (84 %) lesions associated with unstable angina or acute myocardial infarction, compared to 6 of 20 (30 %) lesions with stable angina. Intact vessels devoid of arteriosclerotic disease, such as mammarial arteries and saphenous veins, were without signals for the microorganism (negative controls). Ultrastructurally, chlamydial elementary bodies were found in foam cells and phagocytozing macrophages, also in fragmented extracellular matrix adjacent to apoptotic and necrotic intimal cells. A representative example for chlamydial elementary bodies is illustrated in Figure 1.

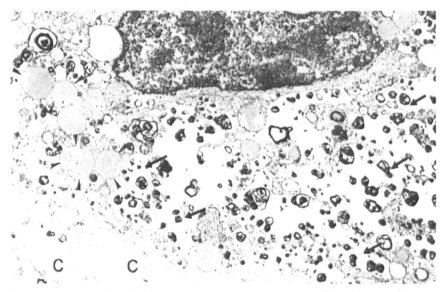

Figure 1. Numerous chlamydial inclusion bodies (arrows) adjacent to a large foam cell in human coronary plaque tissue detected by transmission electron microscopy. Note the large pericellular matrix region filled with lipid vesicles (arrowheads) and chlamydial inclusion bodies, thereby revealing a disintegrated matrix pattern compared to that of neighbored collagen (C)-rich zones; × 11,300.

In conclusion, *C. pneumoniae* were frequently detectable in coronary primary lesions of symptomatic patients. Most importantly, there was a highly significant prevalence of the microorganism in lesions clinically associated with acute coronary syndrome. Predilection sites of *C. pneumoniae* were areas that revealed small healing activity and/or propensity to plaque rupture. The present *in situ* findings indicate a pathogenic role of *Chlamydiae pneumoniae* in human (coronary) plaque rupture.

Discussion

The present study demonstrates that *Chlamydia pneumoniae* is frequently detected in primary coronary atheroma. Our findings are comparable to the results of recent studies on human coronary atherectomy specimens that detected *Chlamydia pneumoniae* in 73 % and 45 %, using immunohistochemistry by a bacterial-specific antibody directed against the *C. pneumoniae* membrane protein OMP1 [12,13]. Certainly, of great importance is our finding of a prevalence of the microorganism in lesions associated with acute coronary syndrome, i.e. unstable angina and acute myocardial infarction, in 84 % compared to lesions with stable angina in 30 %.

In this context, our data demonstrate several predilection sites for *C. pneumoniae*. Predominantly, these are plaque areas with sparse cell density, necrotic areas and regions with neovascularization. Thus, these are intimal areas characterized by a poor healing tendency and/or a propensity to plaque rupture, features that are more frequent in unstable than stable angina lesions [22,23]. Less frequent localizations of *C. pneumoniae* are mural thrombi and ruptured regions, which indicate manifest plaque rupture events or their recent healing. It is of interest that recently we were able to show both programmed and accidental cell death (apoptosis and necrosis) more frequently found in lesions beginning to have unstable angina [19]. Taken together, these findings support the marked prevalence of *C. pneumoniae* in vulnerable atheroma. Also, they point to possible microorganism-induced effects, such as the depletion of smooth muscle cells and/or the disintegration of extracellular matrix that predispose or even lead to the destabilization of (coronary) plaques [4,19].

No signals for *C. pneumoniae* were found in intimal hyperplasia and inflammatory infiltrates, irrespective of the underlying lesion type. As shown by recent investigational work, local cell density in intimal hyperplasia is associated with increased metabolic and matrix secretory activity of smooth muscle cells [20], concordant with growth and a low death rate of these cells [17]. All these events contribute to stabilizing the atheroma's texture. Likewise, the presence of inflammatory infiltrates including lymphocytes suggests a high focal amount of bactericidal activity, such as of interferon-γ [21], and thus the absence of infectious pathogens. Therefore, the absence of *C. pneumoniae* with inflammatory infiltrates and intimal hyperplasia, i.e. with plaque texture features that have healing characteristics, rather supports the concept of *C. pneumoniae*-associated plaque rupture events. Furthermore, importantly, the variant distribution pattern of the microorganism in different plaque areas or lesion types, as found in the present study, argues against the often discussed "innocent bystander" role of *Chlamydia pneumoniae*.

Our observations on human coronary atheroma are confirmed by recent retrospective findings on coronary autopsy material from Alaska inhabitants [24]. These people are generally characterized by a low morbidity due to coronary artery disease. The authors showed that the serologic detection of a *C. pneumoniae* infection (average of 8.7 years pre death of the patients) precedes very often the formation of advanced coronary lesions that harbor the microorganism. Based on these data, for the first time, a pacemaker function in the progression of coronary artery disease has been postulated for chronic chlamydial infections [24]. In addition, a recent study by immunohistochemistry and PCR on 38 autopsy cases demonstrated that *C. pneumoniae* was infrequently (5–13 %) seen in non-cardiovascular tissue such as lung, liver or bone marrow, but was prevalent (29–50 %) in myocardial tissue and in atheroma of central arteries [25]. The authors postulated from their data that the "innocent bystander" hypothesis is not very probable, and also favored the presence of chronic *Chlamydia pneumoniae* infections as the cause for the preferential detection of this pathogen in atheroma of coronary patients.

In summary, present data from our group and others demonstrate that coronary atheroma from symptomatic patients harbor *C. pneumoniae* [12, 13, 18] and thereby suggest that the microorganism contributes to the complication and/or progression of human (coronary) atherosclerosis. Currently, there are ongoing studies in our laboratory that screen for the presence of *Helicobacter pylori* and viruses, such as cytomegalovirus, herpes and Epstein-Barr viruses, in coronary unstable *versus* stable angina atheroma [26].

References

1. Ross R (1999) Atherosclerosis – an inflammatory disease. N Engl J Med 340: 115–126
2. Liuzzo G, Biasucci LM, Gallimore JR, Grillo RL, Rebuzzi AG, Pepys MB, Maseri A (1994) The prognostic value of C-reactive protein and serum amyloid A protein in severe unstable angina. N Engl J Med 331: 417–424
3. Ridker PM, Cushman M, Stampfer MJ, Tracy RP, Hennekens CH (1997) Inflammation, aspirin, and the risk of cardiovascular disease in apparently healthy men. N Engl J Med 336: 973–979
4. Libby P (1995) Molecular bases of acute coronary syndromes. Circulation 91: 2844–2850
5. Libby P, Egan D, Skarlatos S (1997) Roles of infectious agents in atherosclerosis and restenosis. Circulation 96: 4095–4103
6. Danesh J, Collins R, Peto R (1997) Chronic infections and coronary heart disease: is there a link? Lancet 350: 430–436
7. Bauriedel G (1998) Die Arteriosklerose – Abkehr von traditionellen Krankheitstheorien? Herz Kreisl 30: 373–374
8. Kol A, Libby P (1998) The mechanisms by which infectious agents may contribute to atherosclerosis and its clinical manifestations. Trends Cardiovasc Med 8: 191–199
9. Mehta JL, Saldeen TGP, Rand K (1998) Interactive role of infection, inflammation and traditional risk factors in atherosclerosis and coronary artery disease. J Am Coll Cardiol 31: 1217–1225
10. Anderson JL, Carlquist JF, Muhlestein JB, Horne BD, Elmer SP (1998) Evaluation of C-reactive protein, an inflammatory marker, and infectious serology as risk factors for coronary artery disease and myocardial infarction. J Am Coll Cardiol 32: 35–41
11. Marre R, Essig A (1997) *Chlamydia pneumoniae* und Atherosklerose. Dtsch Med Wschr 122: 1092–1095
12. Muhlestein JB, Hammond EH, Carlquist JF, Radicke E, Thomson MJ, Karagounis LA, Woods ML, Anderson JL (1996) Increased incidence of *Chlamydia* species within the coro-

nary arteries of patients with symptomatic atherosclerotic versus other forms of cardiovascular disease. J Am Coll Cardiol 27: 1555–1561
13. Campbell LA, O'Brien ER, Cappuccio AL, Kuo CC, Wang SP, Stewart D, Patton DL, Cummings PK, Grayston JT (1995) Detection of *Chlamydia pneumoniae* TWAR in human coronary atherectomy tissues. J Infect Dis 172: 585–588
14. Saikku P, Mattila K, Nieminen MS, Huttunen JK, Leinonen M, Ekman MR, Mäkelä PH, Valtonen V (1988) Serological evidence of an association of a novel *Chlamydia*, TWAR, with chronic coronary heart disease and acute myocardial infarction. Lancet ii: 983–986
15. Abdelmeguid AE, Ellis SG, Sapp SK, Simpendorfer C, Franco I, Whitlow PL (1994) Directional atherectomy in unstable angina. J Am Coll Cardiol 24: 46–54
16. Braunwald E (1989) Unstable angina. A classification. Circulation 80: 410–414
17. Bauriedel G, Schluckebier S, Hutter R, Welsch U, Kandolf R, Lüderitz B, Forney Prescott M (1998) Apoptosis in restenosis versus stable-angina atherosclerosis. Implications for the pathogenesis of restenosis. Arterioscler Thromb Vasc Biol 18: 1132–1139
18. Bauriedel G, Welsch U, Likungu JA, Welz A, Lüderitz B (1999) *Chlamydia pneumoniae* in koronarem Plaquegewebe: Vermehrter Nachweis bei akutem Koronarsyndrom. Dtsch Med Wschr 124: 375–380
19. Bauriedel G, Hutter R, Welsch U, Bach R, Sievert H, Lüderitz B (1999) Role of smooth muscle cell death in advanced coronary primary lesions: implications for plaque instability. Cardiovasc Res 41: 480–488
20. Bauriedel G, Kandolf R, Schluckebier S, Welsch U (1999) Ultrastructural characteristics of human atherectomy tissue from coronary and lower extremity arterial stenoses. Am J Cardiol 77: 468–474
21. Beatty WL, Morrison RP, Byrne GI (1994) Persistent *Chlamydiae*: from cell culture to a paradigm for chlamydial pathogenesis. Microbiol Rev 58: 686–699
22. Escaned J, van Suylen R, MacLeod DC, Umans VA, de Jong M, Bosman FT, de Feyter PJ, Serruys PW (1993) Histologic characteristics of tissue excised during directional coronary atherectomy in stable and unstable angina pectoris. Am J Cardiol 71: 1442–1447
23. Depré C, Wijns W, Robert AM, Renkin JP, Havaux X (1997) Pathology of unstable plaque: correlation with the clinical severity of acute coronary syndromes. J Am Coll Cardiol 30: 694–702
24. Davidson M, Kuo CC, Middaugh JP, Campbell LA, Wang SP, Newman WP, III, Finley JC, Grayston JT (1998) Confirmed previous infection with *Chlamydia pneumoniae* (TWAR) and its presence in early coronary atherosclerosis. Circulation 98: 628–633
25. Jackson LA, Campbell LA, Schmidt RA, Kuo CC, Cappuccio AL, Lee MJ, Grayston JT (1997) Specificity of detection of *Chlamydia pneumoniae* in cardiovascular atheroma. Am J Pathol 150: 1785–1790
26. Bauriedel G, Hutter R, Lüderitz B (1999) *Chlamydia pneumoniae* and *Helicobacter pylori* in human coronary atherosclerosis. J Am Coll Cardiol 33: 260A–261A
27. Blasi F, Denti F, Erba M, Cosentini R, Raccanelli R, Rinaldi A, Fagetti L, Esposito G, Ruberti U, Allegra L (1996) Detection of *Chlamydia pneumoniae* but not *Helicobacter pylori* in atherosclerotic plaques of aortic aneurysms. J Clin Microbiol 34: 2766–2769
28. Chiu B, Viira E, Tucker W, Fong IW (1997) *Chlamydia pneumoniae*, cytomegalovirus, and herpes simplex virus in atherosclerosis of the carotid artery. Circulation 96: 2144–2148

29. Juvonen J, Laurila A, Juvonen T, Alakärppä H, Surcel HM, Lounatmaa K, Kuusisto J, Saikku P (1997) Detection of *Chlamydia pneumoniae* in human nonrheumatic stenotic aortic valves. J Am Coll Cardiol 29: 1054–1059
30. Kuo CC, Grayston JT, Campbell LA, Goo YA, Wissler RW, Benditt EP (1995) *Chlamydia pneumoniae* (TWAR) in coronary arteries of young adults (15–34 years old). Proc Natl Acad Sci *USA* 92: 6911–6914

3.3.3
Chlamydial lipopolysaccharide and atherosclerosis

H. Brade

On the first slide you see one aspect of LPS which is relevant for all chlamydial diseases. The lipopolysaccharide is the only major surface antigen which represents the whole genus. All the species which were discovered over the years were shown to have one epitope common to all chlamydia, which at the same time has no cross-reactivity with any other lipopolysaccharide or any other natural com-

Epitope specificity of monoclonal antibodies against Chlamydia lipopolysaccharides

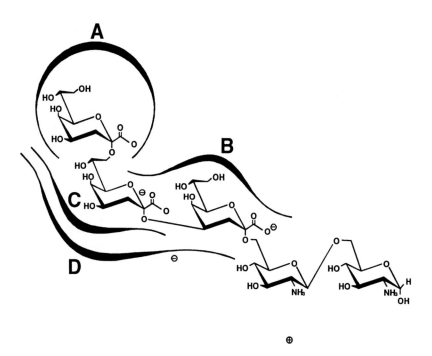

Figure 1. Chemical structure of the carbohydrate backbone of LPS from *C. trachomatis* and schematic representation of monoclonal antibodies binding to distinct Kdo epitopes. Antibodies of type A and B recognize an alpha-pyranosidically linked Kdo monosaccharide residue or the alpha2→4-linked Kdo disaccharide, structures occurring in LPS other than chlamydial. Antibodies of type C and D recognize the disaccharide alpha-Kdo-(2→8)-alpha-Kdo and the trisaccharide alpha-Kdo-(2→8)-alpha-Kdo-(2→4)-alpha-Kdo, respectively. The 2→8-linkage, present in the latter two structures, has not been detected in other bacteria or natural products, and thus, is a chemotaxonomical marker for Chlamydia.

pound. We could clarify this by determining the exact structure of the chlamydia-specific epitope. On the bottom you see the carbohydrate backbone of chlamydial lipopolysaccharide which is composed of two glycosamines belonging to the lipid A moiety which is present in all lipopolysaccharides and anchors the molecule in the outer membrane. Outside of the membrane we have the trisaccharide of Kdo. Within this trisaccharide we see a chemical structure unique in nature: the interlinkage of two Kdo residues by a 2→8 linkage. The presence of this 2→8 linkage is chemically as well as antigenically unique. Antibodies against Kdo in this type of linkage are chlamydia-specific. I have drawn two types, one is the type C antibody for which the disaccharide alone is already enough to confer this Chlamydia specificity, and the type D antibody recognizes the whole molecule.

There are antibodies able to recognize individual Kdo moieties which also occur in other lipopolysaccharides, particularly in enterobacterial lipopolysaccharides, that is for example the type A antibody which binds already to a single terminal Kdo residue, or the type B antibody which recognizes a Kdo disaccharide interlinked by a 2→4 linkage. On top I have drawn the structure of a rough mutant LPS which came out from the mutation of an *E. coli* strain which makes only these two Kdo residues. If you compare these two structures with the antibodies, you see that the type B and A antibodies can bind to these enterobacterial rough mutant LPS as well.

For diagnostic purposes it has often been discussed whether this cross-reactivity may be relevant in making use of these antigens or antibodies in clinical diagnostics. The cross-reactivity is irrelevant under clinical settings. Already the occurrence of rough mutants from normally smooth bacteria is a rather rare event in clinical medicine. These rough mutants always have a complete core, they are deleted only in the genes responsible for the O side chain biosynthesis. I am not aware of any report where under clinical conditions a rough mutant of this type has been isolated from a disease. So with these antibodies you can immediately identify chlamydiae. Whenever you see something staining with this type of antibody, to our present knowledge this is sufficient to diagnose that what you have seen as *Chlamydiae*.

There is another very interesting aspect with this type of molecule. The structure of this epitope was not determined on chlamydial LPS because we did it at a time when we needed quantities, which you could never obtain from naturally grown chlamydiae, for the structural work with conventional biochemical methods by mass spectrometry, by nuclear magnetic resonance. Therefore we took a recombinant approach by cloning a gene-bank from *Chlamydia* into this type of recipients and using monoclonal antibodies of the type C and D as a screening tool. In other words, we cloned the gene responsible to turn an Re-type structure into a chlamydia-type structure. It turned out that this is a Kdo transferase. These transferases are multifunctional enzymes. In *E. coli* a single protein of only 40 kD is able to make two Kdo residues, in *Chlamydia* it is able to make three of them.

In *C. psittaci* it is different. Another message you should take home is that chlamydial LPS is not chlamydial LPS. In *C. psittaci*, in addition to this structure, we get a Kdo trisaccharide of the sequence 2→4–2→4 and a Kdo tetrasaccharide.

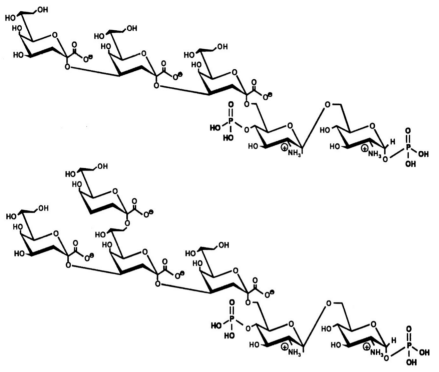

Figure 2. Chemical structures of the carbohydrate backbone of LPS from *C. psittaci* 6BC. The two structures are present in LPS of *C. psittaci* 6BC in addition to the one shown in Figure 1.

Still, *C. psittaci* strains have the epitope located in the trisaccharide you have seen before. Recently, we have generated monoclonal antibodies recognizing these two structures without any cross-reactivity with this structure. Now we have an LPS monoclonal antibody able to differentiate *C. psittaci* from *C. trachomatis*. There is a single report where we, together with the group of Louis de la Maza and Elena Peterson in the US, have studied a monoclonal antibody against *C. pneumoniae* which is able to cross-react at the genus level in immunofluorescence studies but is neutralizing at the species and even at the strain level. So there must be something in *C. pneumoniae* LPS which is not present in all the LPS which we have investigated so far.

A completely different point of view to consider LPS is certainly to look at its endotoxic activity. Most chlamydial infections are characterized by chronic inflammation, and the best example is trachoma. Trachoma is not an infectious disease. The events leading to pannus formation, to vascularization of the cornea are certainly an immunopathological phenomenon going on for a long time without the presence of living microorganisms. This has been known since the late '60s. If we are looking to salpingitis: the primary genital tract infections usually are not causing occluding salpingitis. Repeated genital tract infections obviously sensitize for the development of occluding salpingitis. Many diseases of the lung could be discussed in this context and of course also atherosclerosis, independent of which segment Chlamydia may play a role in. Certainly in all these diseases inflammation is important. If we look to bacterial compounds able to induce a proinflammatory response, there is only one molecule which has all the abilities and which is the best activator of monocytes, endothelial and smooth muscle cells in order to produce proinflammatory cytokines: That is LPS via its endotoxic moiety. Particularly reactive arthritis is a disease you see after gram-negative infection with bacteria having typical endotoxins, whether these are *Shigella*, *Salmonella*, *Yersinia enterocolitica*, *Gonococci* and now, of course, *Chlamydia*.

Negative-ion MALDI-LIN-TOF MS of de-*O*-acylated LPS from *C. trachomatis* L2.

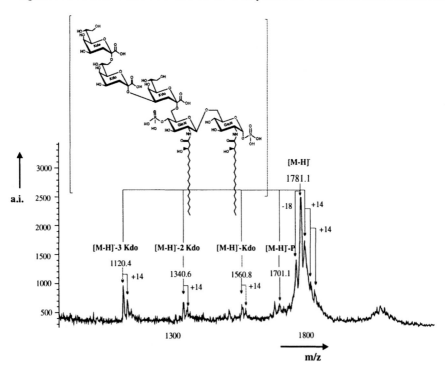

Figure 3. Matrix-assisted laser desorption ionization mass spectrometry (MALDI-MS) of de-O-acylated LPS from *C. trachomatis* L2.

It is quite evident that LPS must play a role as an inducer of proinflammatory response. I was aware of this problem already in '83 or '84. That was our first paper where we checked small quantities of chlamydial LPS in an endotoxin assay system. At that time we were unable to measure cytokines. We were looking for the release of prostaglandines from mouse peritoneal macrophages, for mouse B cell mitogenicity, for toxicity. It was a very poor endotoxin, so I have left this idea behind me for a long time and now we have the data which allow us to clarify the role.

We have now down-scaled our biochemical analytical procedures that we can now work with chlamydial LPS. This is a mass spectrum of chlamydial LPS that is isolated from *C. trachomatis* type L2 where we have removed the ester-linked fatty acids and then we end up with this molecule, and the major peak here is identified as this structure.

Chemical structure of the main molecular species of LPS from *C. trachomatis* L2

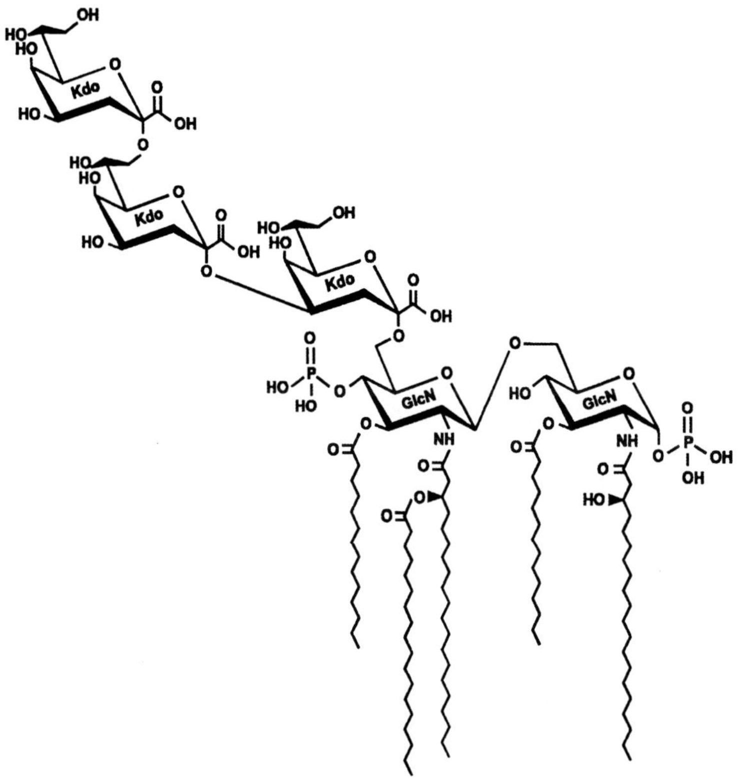

Figure 4. Chemical structure of a major molecular species of LPS from *C. trachomatis* L2. Note that the acyl residues attached to positions 3 and 3' are not hydroxylated.

Now I will show you a summary with many more data where we removed all the fatty acids, the phosphates, and got enough of this type of pentasaccharide to do an NMR analysis on it in order to be able to confirm that the trisaccharide we have seen in recombinant LPS occurs in the same way in *C. trachomatis*. We could also confirm that there is a bisphosphorylated backbone of glucosamine residues but with a significant difference in the acylation pattern compared to typical LPS which we know already. We have access to some 200 to 250 different lipid A structures, and there is one unique feature in chlamydial lipid A: the fatty acids in position 3 and 3' are nonhydroxylated. Since we know that the acylation pattern for example in *E. coli* lipid A can determine whether an endotoxin is an agonist or an antagonist, it certainly could be that chlamydial LPS is composed of a mixture of agonistic and antagonistic molecules which determine their proinflammatory capacity. Since we found that this fatty acid here is only present in half of the molecules, we have a mixture of a tetra- and a penta-acyl species at the ratio of approximately 1:1. The only way how to solve this problem is to synthesize these two types of molecules and the synthesis is finished. The deprotection was done ten days ago, so within the next couple of months we will have the biological data on these two types of molecules and then we can discuss whether chlamydial LPS has agonistic or antagonistic activities.

3.3.4
Clinical trial designs to study antibiotic intervention in atherosclerosis

M. Dunne

A number of lines of evidence point toward an association of *Chlamydia pneumoniae* and atherosclerosis. As evidence of this association mounts, so does an interest in the possibility that antibiotic intervention could ameliorate clinical disease. But when is it justified to start a clinical trial? One first must decide whether sufficient pre-clinical data from either *in vitro* or animal models is available, recognizing that animal models need validation before being considered predictive. Further, a risk/benefit assessment of the safety of the specific intervention must be weighed against the morbidity and mortality of the underlying disease.

Clinical sequelae of atherosclerosis result from peripheral vascular disease, aortic aneurysms, carotid and coronary disease. *C. pneumoniae* has been identified in all of these sites, supporting any one of these patient populations for clinical study. Epidemiologically, coronary artery disease (CAD) produces the greatest burden on society and consequently has been the focus of greatest clinical interest.

True primary prevention of atherosclerosis would be initiated before any clinical evidence of disease is apparent. This group might best benefit from a vaccine approach. Secondary prevention generally refers to prevention of a second myocardial infarction (MI) but could more broadly refer to prevention of ischemic heart disease (IHD). These two groups, post-MI patients and those with evidence of IHD by symptoms or angiographically confirmed, are the target population of a number of ongoing trials. Event rates differ in each of these populations and, coupled with estimated treatment effects, ultimately drive the required sample size of a clinical trial. Careful consideration of both issues is essential to designing a properly powered study that can generate meaningful results.

The events typically considered most definitive include non-fatal myocardial infarction and death, either all cause mortality or are of cardiovascular origin. Recently gaining acceptance has been inclusion of other clinical events related to progression of atherosclerosis such as revascularization procedures and hospitalization for angina. While these latter rates will vary within geographic region, they have been shown to be sensitive markers of underlying disease, correlating with trends in myocardial infarction and death. Addition of these events into a global primary endpoint allows the overall event rates to double and decreases the required sample size by as much as half.

It is not clear how antibiotics could work in this setting. Will they eradicate organisms, fully or partially, and thereby reduce the inflammatory stimulus? Will they simply suppress *C. pneumoniae* while administered and in that way minimize any inflammatory effects? There are few if any good leads to follow, but the underlying suspicion is that longer courses of therapy will be required to have any meaningful effect on this potentially chronic infection.

If *C. pneumoniae* is the agent responsible for some component of an atherosclerotic response, how does one select the population to study? Antibodies are a weak tool for identifying individual patients at risk though they appear to be a marker for associated coronary disease on a population basis. Histologic confirmation is impractical. Culture is much too insensitive. Efforts are underway to assess PCR as a diagnostic tool, but these efforts will need to be validated before general use is appropriate. For now, selectivity on infection status may not be possible.

Table 1: Ongoing trials exploring use of antibiotics as treatment of atherosclerosis.

Trial	Population	Regimen	Size (enrollment)
WIZARD[1]	post-MI	azithro	3,535 (full)
ACES[1]	CAD	azithro	4,000 (open)
MARBLE[1]	CABG-list	azithro	1,200 (open)
STAMINA[2]	peri-MI	anti-HP	600 (open)
APRES[3]	angioplasty	roxithro	1,000 (open)
ANTIBIOS[1]	post-MI	roxithro	4,000 (open)
Munich[4]	angioplasty	roxithro	1,000 (open)

all studies have a placebo arm
azithromycin (azithro) dosing is 600 mg once weekly for 3 months – except ACES which is dosed weekly for one year
STAMINA uses *H. pylori* regimens (PPI/AZ vs AMOX)/MTN)
roxithromycin (roxithro) dosing is 300 mg qd for 4^4–$6^{1,3}$ weeks
WIZARD and ANTIBIOS select on *C. pneumoniae* titer
endpoints: [1]death/MI/revascularization/angina; [2]inflammatory markers; [3,4]restenosis

A number of studies are underway which will aim to identify the risks and benefits of antibiotic intervention in atherosclerosis. These include WIZARD, STAMINA, MARBLE and ACES, using azithromycin, and three other studies using roxithromycin, ANTIBIOS, APRES and an angioplasty trial in Munich. Dosing varies from 4 weeks to one year, but all studies include patients with coronary artery disease. Some use *C. pneumoniae* antibody titers as entry criteria. All use some combination of myocardial infarction, death, revascularization procedures and/or hospitalization for angina or, for post-angioplasty trials, restenosis, as the primary endpoint with follow-up for as long as four years post dosing. Each will offer insight into the possibility of antibiotic intervention in atherosclerosis and, if positive, open a new avenue into treatment for the most significant contributor to morbidity and mortality in Western civilization.

References

1. Shepherd J, Cobbe SM, Ford I, et al. (1995) Prevention of coronary heart disease with pravastatin in men with hypercholesterolemia. N Engl J Med 333 (20): 1300–1307

2. Pedersen TR, Kjekshus J, Berg K, et al. (1994) Randomised trial of cholesterol lowering in 4444 patients with coronary heart disease: the Scandinavian Simvastatin Survival Study (4S). Circulation 344: 1383–1389
3. Sacks FM, Pfeffer MA, Moye LA, et al. (1996) The effect of pravastatin on coronary events after myocardial infarction in patients with average cholesterol levels. N Engl J Med 335 (14): 1001–1009
4. Campbell LA, O'Brien R, Cappuccio AL, Kuo CC, Wang S, Stewart D, Patton DL, Cummings PK, Grayston JT (1995) Detection of *Chlamydia pneumoniae* TWAR in human coronary atherectomy tissues. J Infect Dis 172: 585–588
5. Fong IW, Chiu B, Viira E, Fong MW, Jang D, Mahony J (1997) Rabbit Model for *Chlamydia pneumoniae* Infection. JCM 35: 48–52
6. Laitinen K, Alakarppa H, Laurila A, Leinonen M (1997) Animal models for *Chlamydia pneumonia* infection. Scand J Infect Dis 104 (Suppl): 15–17
7. Dunne MW (1998) The Association of *Chlamydia pneumoniae* and Atherogenesis. In: Scheld WM, Craig WA, Hughes JM (eds.), Emerging Infections (2. ed.). ASM Press

Discussion

Bhakdi:
Are the patients getting statins ?

Dunne:
Yes, all patients in these studies get optimal medical care. This will be important because you really need to see whether an antibiotic adds any additional benefit to what we already know about the treatment of their particular problems. But just on that point, it is interesting that we now have 2 or 3 studies which show mortality advantages for people on statins in a variety of different settings such as post-myocardial infarction, even at normal cholesterol. But in clinical practice in the US only about a third of patients who are eligible and appropriate for statins are actually getting them. I am not as clear as what is happening outside the US.

Stille:
It can be debated if in the WIZARD study and in all the other studies they have the right dosage for the antibiotics. In our opinion the dosage is critically low. For studies in Germany we take higher doses of azithromycin while we recommend a shorter duration, two months, but with these higher dosages, with the conventional standard dosage of 500 mg. Your recommendation is below the official standard doses of azithromycin, so there is a risk that maybe the WIZARD study, and all the other studies that follow the WIZARD model, will lead to a negative result due to a wrong dosage.

Dunne:
That is possible. Let me ask you a follow-up question: the recommended dose of azithromycin for which indication?

Stille:
For respiratory tract infection.

Dunne:
The dose of azithromycin in general respiratory infections is based more on extracellular levels of azithromycin in relation to coverage of *Streptococcus pneumoniae* than it is for coverage of an intracellular organism such as *Chlamydia pneumoniae*. The dose for *Chlamydia trachomatis* urethritis is only 1 g, given as a single dose. That is not the approved dose for respiratory tract infections, but at this lower dose it still has efficacy. Dosing in the WIZARD study actually had the 'respiratory tract' course of drug to start with, specifically 600 mg a day for 3 days, which is initially more than the RTI dose. So the initial treatment should cover whatever the general RTI dose covers. The dose in the WIZARD study is longer than three days in order to better treat an infection that can persist in a latent state for prolonged periods of time.

We have given a 1200 mg dose once a week for prophylaxis of *Mycobacterium avium* infection (MAC) in AIDS patients, and that is an approved dose. The MIC_{90} for MAC is 32 µg/ml, not 0.2 µg/ml as it is for *C. pneumoniae*. The difficulty with a 1200 mg per week dose is that you are going to get GI intolerance in the long run which in this population may not be as well tolerated as in the HIV population. So there were trade-offs made. We do have some sense that a weekly dose in this range will work to prevent an intracellular infection. It is possible that we have not chosen the correct dose but it appeared to be the best option.

Marre:
Microbiologists are always afraid of resistance development when antibiotics are given in large scale. Is it planned that antibiotic resistance of the oral flora is monitored too in this trial?

Dunne:
We had discussions internally on this topic during the design of the protocol. Essentially, the use of any antibiotic has the potential to alter the normal flora. This change could be seen with short or long courses of antibiotics. A study has been performed recently by Heppner, published in *Clinical Infectious Diseases*, in which throat swabs were taken of military recruits who received a weekly 500 mg dose for three months. At the end of the dosing interval, there was no significant increase in the distribution of resistant *S. pneumoniae* compared to baseline. At least in that experience, there seemed to be no major impact of a three-month course of antibiotics on the development of resistance.

Even so, it is possible that there will be a change in the percentage of resistant organisms in the colonizing flora of patients who receive this chronic course of therapy. We had considered adding a throat swab to this protocol but it was logistically infeasible. We are collecting the incidence of any bacterial infections that occur at any time during the period of observation. We have also requested that any bacteria isolated during these events be sent to a central lab for sensitivity testing. However, given that many of these investigators are cardiologists and that these infections will be treated by the primary caregiver, it may be difficult to obtain many organisms. But, as you know, the morbidity and mortality associated with atherosclerosis is very large. The risk/benefit assessment of antibiotic use in the treatment of atherosclerosis will need to factor the impact of cardiovascular protection with other costs associated with treatment.

Byrne:

You mentioned that optimally you might only be showing efficacy against some proportion of the population that you are dealing with. Are you set up to look at subgroups afterwards and how are you going to deal with them?

Dunne:

We have an extensive screening questionnaire that provides information regarding the patients' medical history. Subgroups, based on medical history, can be assessed to explore who may have experienced the most benefit. We have also banked serology from numerous trial visits. Some testing is being done while the trial is ongoing. Other serology will be stored for future use to explore various inflammatory markers. We will not be able to run PCR assays from the WIZARD population as we have not banked any cells.

Bhakdi:

The resistance problem is really very important and in my opinion the helicobacter problem is much more pressing than taking throat swabs. Every second person in the world has helicobacter and the monotherapy with the macrolide is, as we all know, a mistake. Are we going to take this risk? You are willing to do a monotherapy on 10,000 people of which 5,000 have helicobacter, and you cannot check for the resistance of helicobacter that may emerge. I come from Thailand and I know that we have a lot of helicobacter resistance because you get macrolides across the counter.

Dunne:

Yes, that could be an issue. The efficacy of a 600 mg single tablet against *H. pylori* will be a range of about 5 %. We have done that study. The likelihood is that the vast majority of the helicobacter colonies will not be impacted. But if your point is that some fraction of the helicobacter could be impacted by this treatment, that this is something we will have to continue to consider.

Kreuz:

A standard criterion for assessment of efficacy, the dose relationship, is a very important factor. As far as I understood, at this moment no efforts are made to get data on the dosage/efficacy relationship.

Dunne:

We had a dose response protocol on the table initially, but we would have been required to take significance adjustments for multiple comparisons. We were up to about 8,500 people just to do two doses plus placebo. It became something we just can't focus on right now. The best dose response that we will have for now will be the ACES compared with the WIZARD study. This comparison will give you a sense of whether or not there is a dramatic improvement with longer dosing. Once we know the treatment effect of the intervention, we may be able to bring the total numbers of enrolled subjects down and we can start doing additional trials to get at that question.

Bauriedel:

May I ask you about your inclusion criteria in the WIZARD study? You told us that these patients had already had an infarction. Are they still symptomatic, are they even unstable or is the only criterion that they have had an infarction?

Dunne:

That criterion, how long after their infarction patients should wait to be eligible for enrollment, was discussed many times. We brought it back to six weeks after their infarction because in looking at how people do post infarction, by about 6 weeks after the event rate is almost approaching what it is chronically. The median post-MI time in the study is about two years. So they are really well out from their original MI.

3.3.5
Why antibiotics against *Chlamydia pneumoniae* for treatment of atherosclerotic disease could fail

J.M. Ossewaarde

I will show you some data that might suggest that antibiotic treatment could fail for the treatment of *C. pneumoniae* in atherosclerotic lesions. First of all when you summarize the literature there is a striking discrepancy between PCR and immunocytochemistry results. We have summarized here 12 studies of 239 patients in which both PCR and ICC were used on the material of the same patient (Figure 1). What you see if you use a gold standard of either positive in PCR or immunocytochemistry, then PCR alone detects only 50 % of all the patients having *C. pneumoniae* and immunocytochemistry detects over 80 %. Usually PCR is considered a much more sensitive technique than immunocytochemistry. So why is PCR less sensitive than immunocytochemistry?

Today only 13 isolates have been obtained of 224 reported attempts. I am sure there are many hundreds more attempts that are negative for isolation of *C. pneumoniae*. There are also some other studies in which *C. pneumoniae* DNA could not be detected in atherosclerotic lesions (Figure 2). However, that is only failure to detect DNA of *C. pneumoniae*. These authors did not consider the possibility of the presence of chlamydial antigens.

We have studied this discrepancy in some more detail. I will show you some data of animal model studies we have done on lung infections in mice. We have examined the lungs 2 days after infection and 21 days after infection by a whole series of techniques detecting antigens or detecting 16S rRNA. When we look at these *in situ* techniques, we see two types of staining: a granular staining and a compact staining that resembles inclusions you also see when you use cell monolayers *in vitro*, very compact inclusions which are always positive with all techniques, antigen detection techniques and RNA as well as DNA detection techniques. We have a granular type of staining pattern which is only positive for antigens and we see this granular type of staining in macrophages. Sometimes macrophages have compact inclusions but not that many. Later on in infection we usually see only granular staining in macrophages and hardly any compact inclusions. Compact inclusions are also positive for RNA, and granular staining is always only positive for antigen and negative for RNA and DNA (Figure 3).

I will show you some examples. This is a section of a lung of a mouse two days after infection, and this is *in situ* hybridization using an oligonucleotide for dissection as RNA of *C. pneumoniae*. You see very nice and clear inclusions in epithelial cells.

This is a mouse lung 21 days after infection (Figure 4), we see the bronchus-associated lymphoid tissue and positive cells, probably macrophages, which show a staining pattern dispersed throughout the cell, not confined to a typical inclusion. It has a granular aspect which you can see much better if you are working with the microscope yourself. This is actually Chlamydia heat-shock protein 60 which is positive in this section, but also RR402 and anti-LPS antibodies are positive. In these cells DNA and RNA are nearly always negative.

Summary of findings: we have studied human specimens from abdominal aneurysms, carotid stenosis (obtained by surgery) and carotid arteries (obtained by autopsy) with Type I and II lesions and more advanced lesions. Membrane protein detected by RR402 is detected in almost all cases, in aneurysms in 100 % and in advanced cases of carotis arteries in 100 % and half of the cases of carotis stenoses. LPS detection is very variable, it depends on the hybridoma we used for these assays and ranged between 32 and over 70 %. If you add them all together, about 80 % are positive.

Hsp60 was only present in a few specimens in surgically obtained carotid stenosis specimens and not in the other specimens. We could not find any DNA or RNA, DNA not by PCR and not by *in situ* hybridization, RNA not by *in situ* hybridization (Figure 5).

So what do we see? In *in vitro* infected cells we always have clearly visible inclusions, compact staining positive in all techniques, in animal specimens early in infection we see clearly visible inclusions. Later in infection we see granular staining throughout the cytoplasm and do not see any clearly visible inclusions, while in human specimens we observe only the granular stainings throughout the cytoplasm and no clearly visible inclusions (Figure 6). Since there is no DNA and RNA present anymore, we think that those bacteria are no longer viable and hence not susceptible to antibiotics anymore.

What can antibiotics do when you give them to patients with atherosclerosis? They have several side effects which can be a problem when you want to analyze antibiotic trials. Tetracyclines inhibit metalloproteinases and they have also shown to be effective in reducing the risk for aneurysms, and macrolides have various antiinflammatory effects. I have listed some of them here and they can all confound your results of antibiotic trials. You have to take these into consideration (Figure 7).

		PCR		ICC	
		+	−	+	−
PCR or ICC	+	65	59	103	21
	−	0	115	0	115
Sensitivity		52.4%		83.1%	

Based on 239 patients in 12 studies

PCR + ICC positive in ~ 50%
Isolation positive in only 13 of 224 reported attempts

Figure 1. Discrepancies in detection of *Chlamydia pneumoniae*.

Failure to detect *Chlamydia pneumoniae* in coronary atheromas of patients undergoing atherectomy.	Weiss et al., 1996
Failure to demonstrate *Chlamydia pneumoniae* in symptomatic abdominal aortic aneurysms by a nested polymerase chain reaction (PCR).	Lindholt et al., 1998
Failure to detect *Chlamydia pneumoniae* in atherosclerotic plaques of Australian patients.	Paterson et al., 1998
Failure to detect *Chlamydia pneumoniae* in calcific and degenerative arteriosclerotic aortic valves excised during open heart surgery.	Andreasen et al., 1998

Figure 2. *Chlamydia pneumoniae* DNA not always detected.

	Time after intranasal infection			
	2 days		21 days	
	antigen	16S rRNA	antigen	16S rRNA
bronch./alv. epithelial cells	++	++	−	−
macrophages	++ granular staining	+ compact inclusions	+ granular staining	± compact inclusions

±: sporadic positive cells; +: few positive cells; ++: many positive cells

Figure 3. Animal model time series of *Chlamydia pneumoniae*.

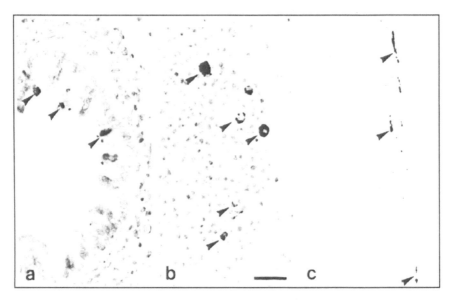

Figure 4. *Chlamydia pneumoniae* in situ: a) mouse lung epithelium, b) mouse lung BALT, c) human atherosclerotic tissue.

	Abdominal aneurysms	Carotid stenosis	Carotid arteries Type I–II	Carotid arteries Type IV–VI
membrane protein	100%	50%	0%	100%
LPS	32–74%	22%	0%	83%
hsp60	0%	17%	0%	0%
DNA	0%	0%	0%	0%
rRNA	ND	0%	0%	0%
Number	19	18	7	6

Figure 5. Presence of *Chlamydia pneumoniae* in human specimens.

In *in vitro* infected cells:
        clearly visible inclusions
        compact staining

In animal lung specimens:
    early in infection:
        clearly visible inclusions
        compact staining
    late in infection:
        granular throughout the cytoplasm
        no clearly visible inclusions

In human specimens:
        granular throughout the cytoplasm
        no clearly visible inclusions

Figure 6. Aspect of staining of *Chlamydia pneumoniae*.

Tetracyclines	inhibit metallo-proteinases
Macrolides Roxithromycin Azithromycin Clarithromycin Erythromycin	anti-inflammatory, affect migration of neutrophils, affect oxidative burst in phagocytes, affect production of cytokines, neutrophil membrane stabilizing interaction, induce neutrophil apoptosis

Figure 7. Possible confounding effects of antibiotics in atherosclerosis.

3.3.6
Atherosclerosis: Why the search for a causative infectious agent is not warranted

S. Bhakdi

The author contends that there is sufficient evidence to exclude a major causative role for infectious agents in the pathogenesis of atherosclerosis. The arguments are summarized as follows.

Each LDL molecule is itself endowed with the potential to be transformed into an atherogenic molecule, in the absence of oxidation or infection. LDL can be converted to a *quasi*-infectious agent that activates complement and macrophages, the archaic components of our immune system. Atherosclerosis is proposed to represent a novel form of an immunological disease that is triggered and sustained by unhalted activation of these effector systems [1].

Transformation of LDL to its atherogenic derivative occurs when the lipoprotein is stranded in tissues, i.e. in the subendothelial space of arteries. Transformation occurs by degradation of the lipoprotein particle by enzymes that are probably ubiquitously present in connective tissues. This contention is supported by the following experimental evidence.

1. Treatment of LDL with degrading (but non-oxidizing) enzymes converts the molecule *in vitro* to a pro-inflammatory moiety [2]. Other lipoproteins cannot be transformed in the same manner. Degraded (but not oxidized) LDL triggers inflammation via two independent but converging pathways. First, enzymatically degraded LDL (E-LDL) binds C-reactive protein (CRP), and this causes activation of the classical complement pathway [3]. Furthermore, exposure of unesterified cholesterol in the degraded lipoprotein causes activation of the alternative complement pathway [2]. Second, E-LDL causes upregulation of adhesion molecules on endothelial cells and promotes transmigration of monocytes [4]. E-LDL is then rapidly taken up by macrophages, inducing foam cell formation [2]. Macrophage foam cells synthesize and secrete a specific spectrum of cytokines, of which macrophage chemotactic protein (MCP-1) dominates. At higher concentrations, E-LDL also induces production of small quantities of IL-6 and promotes apoptosis [5]. In contrast, neither IL-1β- nor IL-8- or TNF-α-secretion is enhanced by E-LDL. It is of distinct interest that macrophage activation by E-LDL differs fundamentally from their activation by microorganisms including Chlamydia. The specific spectrum of cytokines induced by E-LDL explains why the atherosclerotic lesion does not display the typical pathology of an acute (purulent) or chronic (granulomatous) bacterial infection.
2. The *in vitro* findings have *in vivo* correlates. E-LDL, CRP and activated complement components are always present in atherosclerotic lesions [3,6–8]. C5b-9 deposition correlates temporally with lipid deposition, occurring even

before monocytes infiltrate the lesions [9]. E-LDL has been detected by immunohistochemistry by using specific monoclonal antibodies in all early human lesions and in co-localization with CRP [7]. Such extensive deposition of complement in the atherosclerotic lesions would not be explainable by the presence of small numbers of Chlamydia in a fraction of the lesions. E-LDL has also been isolated from human lesions and shown to activate complement [6].

The E-LDL hypothesis contends that conversion of the lipoprotein to its degraded derivative in the subendothelium is the sole process that is required to trigger atherogenesis. E-LDL will bind CRP, activate complement, attract monocyte-macrophages, and thus promote its own uptake and clearance from the vessel wall. HDL assumes a central function because it promotes reverse cholesterol transport from the foam cells. Through these mechanisms, small amounts of stranded LDL are continuously being cleared from connective tissues. Elevated plasma LDL levels will, however, increase the amount of trapped lipoproteins, and any damage to the endothelium will augment this process. In the face of excessive foam cell formation, cytotoxic and proinflammatory processes gain dominance, and the LDL removal process acquires a negative, pathological aspect. Lipid-release from dead foam cells sustain a vicious circle of events, which is driven by the unhalted activation of complement and macrophages [1].

Thus, atherosclerosis may be viewed as a novel type of immunological disease that is caused by excessive trapping of LDL in the subendothelium. Three predictions emerge from the concept: (1) suppression of complement or macrophage activation should counteract atherogenesis; (2) *vice versa*, priming or overactivation of complement and monocytes-macrophages should promote atherogenesis; (3) lowering of LDL plasma levels below a critical threshold should reduce trapping of the lipoprotein to an extent that abolishes atherogenesis.

All three predictions have essentially been fulfilled. (1) We have shown that a defect in the terminal complement sequence protects against diet-induced atherosclerosis in rabbits [10]. These results highlight the hitherto unappreciated fact that complement is indeed of central importance in atherogenesis. (2) We have found that application of pure endotoxin markedly enhances atherogenesis. Cholesterol-fed rabbits that were given intravenous injections of endotoxin once a week developed much more extensive lesions than did the controls (unpublished data). Hence, it is apparent that **any** exaggerated activation of the unspecific immune system will promote atherogenesis, irrelevant of the site of infection, and there appears no valid reason to assume that *vascular* infections should be of particular importance. (3) Clinical trials have amply documented the efficacy of lipid lowering agents (statins) in the prevention of coronary heart disease [11]. Of importance, lowering LDL levels also leads to *regression* of atherosclerotic lesions, *in the absence of any antibiotic treatment* [12]. Thus, as with a genuine infectious disease, elimination of the causative agent – in this case tissue-deposited E-LDL – prevents and heals the disease.

In the face of this evidence, we are bound by duty to propagate *established* effective measures to combat this major disease of industrialized nations. The means are already at our disposal. It is not contested that Chlamydia may be present in some atherosclerotic lesions; however, since the pathologic processes can be halted and even be induced to regress without any anti-infective measure, a significant causative role of infectious agents is most improbable. Antibiotic therapy of atherosclerosis is not only unnecessary, but represents an unwarranted hazard to the patient and to the population in general.

It is the author's view that the arguments **for** a role of *Chlamydia pneumoniae* in atherogenesis are warped by bias, and a critical appraisal of any claim will reveal its weaknesses. A few examples follow.

1. Serological findings are widely cited in support of the Chlamydia hypothesis. However, it is now apparent that there is no correlation between antibody titers and the presence of Chlamydia in atherosclerotic lesions [13], and consequently there is no basis for the assumption that elevated antibody titers against *C. pneumoniae* arise from vascular infections.
2. Although it is claimed that antibiotic treatment of patients with coronary disease is beneficial, this statement is not supported by a single well-conducted placebo-controlled trial.
3. An immunopathological response to Chlamydia can cause myocarditis [14], and this finding is being cited as support for the chlamydial genesis of atherosclerosis. However, myocarditis and atherosclerosis are two unrelated diseases. It is furthermore worthy of note that the pathology described in the *Science* paper was invoked by *C. trachomatis*, whereas *C. pneumoniae* was not effective!
4. Another paper claims to show that exaggeration of atherosclerotic lesions in cholesterol-fed mice was invoked by *C. pneumoniae*, whereas *C. trachomatis* was not effective [15]. However, the dose of *C. pneumoniae* used in that study was 1000-fold higher than the dose of *C. trachomatis*, so the conclusion reached by the authors clearly does not follow.

Overall, therefore, the **pro** discussions are not being conducted in a stringent and scholarly fashion. This must be a cause of deep concern.

References

1. Bhakdi S (1998) Complement and atherogenesis: the unknown connection. Ann Med 30: 503–507
2. Bhakdi S, Dorweiler B, Kirchmann R, Torzewski J, Weise E, Tranum-Jensen J, Walev I, Wieland E (1995) On the pathogenesis of atherosclerosis: enzymatic transformation of human low density lipoprotein to an atherogenic moiety. J Exp Med 182: 1959–1971
3. Bhakdi S, Torzewski M, Klouche M, Hemmes M (1999) Complement and atherogenesis: binding of CRP to degraded, non-oxidized LDL enhances complement activation. Arterioscler Thromb Vasc Biol 19: 2348–2354
4. Klouche M, May AE, Hemmes M, Messner M, Kanse SM, Preissner K, Bhakdi S (1999) Enzymatically modified, non-oxidized LDL induces selective adhesion and transmigration

of monocytes and T-lymphocytes through human endothelial cell monolayers. Arterioscler Thromb Vasc Biol 19: 784–793
5. Klouche M, Gottschling S, Gerl V, Hell W, Husmann M, Dorweiler B, Messner M, Bhakdi S (1998) Atherogenic properties of enzymatically degraded LDL: selective induction of MCP-1 and cytotoxic effects on human macrophages. Arterioscler Thromb Vasc Biol 18: 1376–1385
6. Seifert PS, Hugo F, Tranum-Jensen J, Zahringer U, Muhly M, Bhakdi S (1990) Isolation and characterization of a complement-activating lipid extracted from human atherosclerotic lesions. J Exp Med 172: 547–557
7. Torzewski M, Klouche M, Hock J, Messner M, Dorweiler B, Torzewski J, Gabbert HE, Bhakdi S (1998) Immunohistochemical demonstration of enzymatically modified human LDL and its colocalization with the terminal complement complex in the early atherosclerotic lesion. Arterioscler Thromb Vasc Biol 18: 369–378
8. Torzewski J, Torzewski M, Bowyer DE, Fröhlich M, Koenig W, Waltenberger J, Fitzsimmons C, Hombach V (1998) C-reactive protein frequently colocalizes with the terminal complement complex in the intima of early atherosclerotic lesions of human coronary arteries. Arterioscler Thromb Vasc Biol 18: 1386–1392
9. Seifert PS, Hugo F, Hansson GK, Bhakdi S (1989) Prelesional complement activation in experimental atherosclerosis. Terminal C5b-9 complement deposition coincides with cholesterol accumulation in the aortic intima of hypercholesterolemic rabbits. Lab Invest 60: 747–754
10. Schmiedt W, Kinscherf R, Deigner HP, Kamencic H, Nauen O, Kilo J, Oelert H, Metz J, Bhakdi S (1998) Complement C6-deficiency protects against diet-induced atherosclerosis in rabbits. Arterioscler Thromb Vasc Biol 18: 1790–1795
11. Hebert PR, Gaziano JM, Chan KS, Hennekens H (1997) Cholesterol lowering with statin drugs, risk of stroke, and total mortality. J Am Med Ass 278: 313–320
12. de Groot E, Jukema JW, van Swijjndregt ADM, Zwinderman AH, Ackerstaff RGA, van der Steen AFW, Bom N, Lie KI, Bruschke VG (1998) B-mode ultrasound assessment of pravastatin treatment effect on carotid and femoral artery walls and its correlations with coronary arteriographic findings: a report of the regression growth evaluation statin study (REGRESS). J Am Coll Cardiol 31: 1561–1567
13. Maass M, Gieffers J, Krause E, Engel PM, Bartels C, Solbach W (1998) Poor correlation between microimmunofluorescence serology and polymerase chain reaction for detection of vascular *Chlamydia pneumoniae* infection in coronary artery disease patients. Med Microbiol Immunol 187: 1103–1106
14. Bachmaier K, Neu N, de la Maza LM, Pal S, Hessel A, Penninger JM (1999) *Chlamydia* infections and heart disease linked through antigenic mimicry. Science 283: 1335–1339
15. Hu H, Pierce GN, Zongh G (1999) The atherogenic effects of chlamydia are dependent on serum cholesterol and specific to *Chlamydia pneumoniae*. J Clin Invest 103: 747–753

3.4
Chlamydia infections and arthritis

J. Sieper

Reactive arthritis (ReA) or arthritis in general is much more frequently associated with *C. trachomatis* than *C. pneumoniae*. I will briefly introduce you to the clinical picture of reactive arthritis. Reactive arthritis occurs after urogenital tract infection with Chlamydia and the symptoms normally occur days or weeks after the initial infection. Often – as you also know from *C. pneumoniae* – the initiating infection is asymptomatic. Chlamydial antigen, DNA and even RNA have been found in the joint, making it very likely that Chlamydia survive in the joint. One of the pioneers who looked for DNA and RNA has been Alan Hudson who today presents the data on Alzheimer disease. A very similar clinical picture can be seen after gut infections with enterobacteria, and some of the data I will present for *C. trachomatis* also include data from *Yersinia*- and *Salmonella*-induced reactive arthritis.

It just happens that in ReA the knee-joint is often involved which makes it relatively easy to obtain synovial fluid for further investigation and also synovial membrane for studies.

Nonetheless, a few years ago we have described 5 patients with reactive arthritis after a preceding infection with *C. pneumoniae* and the clinical picture is quite similar. Knee, elbow and wrist joints are involved. The preceding symptoms were pharyngitis, bronchitis or no symptoms at all before the arthritis occurred. The arthritis was often self limiting with a duration of one month, two months or a few days [1].

I will present the typical case of a patient who had a bronchitis one week before he came to our clinic at day 7 with a gonarthritis. At day 7 the antibodies against *C. pneumoniae* were negative and there was a gradual increase to a highly positive titer over the next days and weeks. These titers were done by John Treharne years ago by microimmuno-fluorescence. We also had the opportunity to investigate synovial fluid of this patient several times because he had a relapsing infusion in the knee joint, and we stimulated the T-cells from synovial fluid with different antigens. There was some cross-reactivity in the T-cell-response to both types of Chlamydia, but there was a higher response to *C. pneumoniae*, while this difference was not so clear in the peripheral blood. Therefore *C. pneumoniae* can also cause arthritis and there have been some reports on the detection of *C. pneumoniae* in the joint in patients with arthritis. We have reported one patient [2], and then Alan Hudson has reported that in a relatively unselected group of patients with different forms of arthritis *C. trachomatis* could be detected ten times more frequently than *C. pneumoniae*. In another study we were involved in and which was conducted in Michael Ward's lab in Southampton we found *C. trachomatis* in 28 % of patients with arthritis of unknown origin, while none of these patients were positive for *C. pneumoniae* [6].

The conclusion from this is that *C. pneumoniae* can lead to a form of reactive arthritis but not frequently, and that *C. trachomatis* is a much more frequent cause of arthritis. This might be related to the site of the bacterial entrance. As I told you before, you get also reactive arthritis after gut infections. The lower part of the body might therefore be connected to this form of arthritis, while a bacterial entrance via the lung might not so easily get access to these joints. This is just a speculation, I do not have a better explanation at the moment.

There are quite a few studies that *C. trachomatis* play an important role for arthritis. There were studies from Geneva, from Alan Hudson's lab and from our patients [6] that in about 30 % of patients with an undifferentiated oligoarthritis (an arthritis without other explanation) *C. trachomatis* can be found in the joints. If you look in synovial membrane – again from Philadelphia – the detection level is even higher in a similar group of patients where they found 30 % of patients being positive in synovial fluid, but 50 % in synovial membrane.

The question is why Chlamydia persists *in vivo*, and we have tried to address this question. I will present some data from our studies in Chlamydia-induced arthritis and I think that some conclusion can be drawn which might be also true for infections with *C. pneumoniae*.

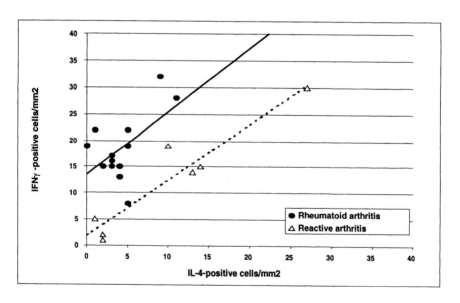

Figure 1. A higher number IFN-γ- than IL-4-positive cells are found in the synovial membrane of rheumatoid arthritis (RA) patients in comparison to those with reactive arthritis (ReA). Synovial tissue from 12 patients with RA and 7 patients with ReA was stained and cytokine-positive cells were counted as described in the Methods section. The line shows the linear regression for RA patients and the dotted line for ReA patients. (with permission of *Rheumatology*, see ref. # 9)

For those of you who are not so familiar with this concept I will give a brief introduction to T-helper 1 (TH1) and TH2 cells. These cells have been known now for about 12 years. TH1 cells secrete IFN-γ, and in this context TNF-α probably is also very important. For the elimination of many bacteria you need TH1 cells with the production of IFN-γ and maybe a primary or secondary production of TNF-α to kill bacteria such as Chlamydia. In contrast, TH2 cells produce IL-4 and IL-10, and these cytokines are known to inhibit such a response and the fight against intracellular bacteria. There have been quite a few papers now clearly showing that TH1 cytokines are protective in animal models against *C. trachomatis* and I think also against *C. pneumoniae*, and if you add IL-10 or if you have too much IL-10, this leads to a persistence and to a higher number of Chlamydia *in vivo*. Therefore we asked whether an imbalance of the cytokine pattern in reactive arthritis could partly explain why some patients with Chlamydia infections get arthritis and some do not [5].

Figure 1 shows the ratio of IFN-γ-/IL-4-positive cells in the synovial membrane of seven patients with reactive arthritis. We compared these to patients with rheumatoid arthritis which is a completely different disease with a different pathogenesis. Rheumatoid arthritis is believed to be an autoimmune disease. As you can see from Figure 1, the ratio of IFN-γ-/IL-4-positive cells is indeed lower in reactive arthritis compared to rheumatoid arthritis [9].

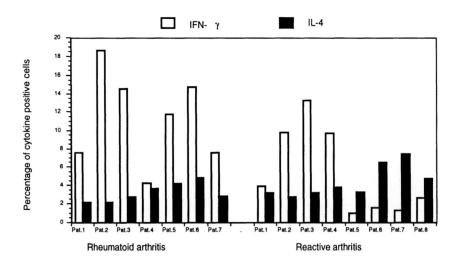

Figure 2. Two color immunofluorescence of gated CD4+ lymphocytes for IFN-γ and IL-4 expression in rheumatoid arthritis (RA) and reactive arthritis (ReA). Synovial fluid mononuclear cells (MNC) were stimulated with anti-CD3 and anti-CD28 in the presence of Monensin and stained as described in the Method section. CD4+ T were gated and quadrant markers were positioned to include >99 of isotype-matched Ig staining cells in the lower left quadrant. (with permission of *Rheumatology*, see ref. # 9)

We also investigated synovial fluid T-cells taken from patients with reactive arthritis compared to rheumatoid arthritis, which were analyzed by intracellular cytokine staining and quantified by flow cytometry. This is a more accurate method than using the microscope and counting the cells by eye. You can see from Figure 2 that the ratio of IFN-γ-/IL-4-positive cells is again higher in rheumatoid arthritis than in reactive arthritis [9]. We also investigated synovial fluid T-cells from 9 patients with reactive arthritis and stimulated these T-cells with *C. trachomatis*. In all these patients it was clear that this was the triggering antigen, and as you can see these patients make a lot of IL-10 and a relatively small amount of TNF-α [7]. We compared this to patients with Lyme arthritis in whom we also investigated synovial fluid T-cells which were stimulated *in vitro* by *Borrelia burgdorferi* antigen [8]. The IL-10/IFN-γ ratio and even more the IL-10/IFN-α ratio were clearly higher compared to Lyme arthritis.

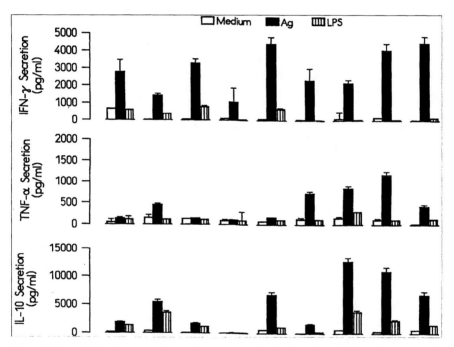

Figure 3. Synovial fluid mononuclear cells were stimulated with whole Chlamydia antigen (Ag) medium alone or lipopolysaccharide (LPS). Cytokines were determined after 48 hours in the supernatant. (with permission of *Arthritis & Rheumatism*, see ref. # 7)

Finally, we investigated 53 patients with early reactive arthritis and compared these to different control groups [3]. We took peripheral blood mononuclear cells from patients with a disease duration of less than 8 weeks. T-cells were stimulated with PHA and the cytokine secretion was analyzed in the supernatant. In this study the level of TNF-α was lower in ReA compared to early (<6 months) rheumatoid arthritis (Figure 3).

We then took the same patient cohort and divided them into two groups: patients with an extended disease (disease duration of longer than 6 months) compared to those with a limited disease (disease duration shorter than 6 months). As you can see from Figure 4, the TNF-α level was lower in patients with longer disease duration compared to those with a shorter disease duration. We also did cytokine analysis at different time points, and the most consistent result was that there was a good correlation between chronic disease courses and a low TNF-α level. Thus a low TNF-α level correlated well with the chronicity in reactive arthritis.

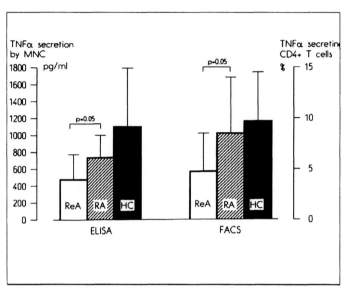

Figure 4. Reactive arthritis (ReA) patients secreted less TNF-α than rheumatoid arthritis (RA) patients. A (left axis): Comparison of the initial TNF-α secretion of peripheral blood mononuclear cells (MNC) upon mitogen stimulation measured by ELISA (see Methods) in 53 patients with ReA and 30 patients with RA. B: (right axis): Comparison of 12 ReA with 12 RA patients for the percentage of TNF-α-positive CD4 T cells (for details see Methods). (with permission of *Arthritis & Rheumatism*, see ref. # 3)

Summarizing this part of our investigation, we believe that in reactive arthritis there is indeed a relative deficiency of important cytokines such as IFN-γ and – which might be even more important – of TNF-α, and that relatively more IL-10 and maybe also IL-4 might be present which allows a persistence of bacteria. We have not worked out yet the relative contribution of these four cytokines, but we will continue to study this subject and I think, summarizing our whole data, that TNF-α and IL-10 might be the key players.

Here are results from the antibiotic trial we performed in about 100 patients with reactive arthritis or possible reactive arthritis. Half of the patients were treated with Ciprofloxacin for three months and the other half were treated with

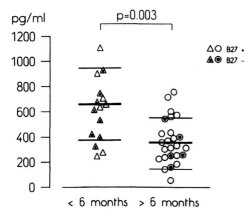

Figure 5. Comparison of the initial TNF-α secretion by peripheral blood mononuclear cells upon mitogen stimulation measured by ELISA (see Methods) in 40 patients with reactive arthritis (ReA), divided into two groups according to their disease duration: $\geq$ 6 months, n=15) or <6 months, n=25). ReA patients with longer disease duration secreted less TNF-α than ReA patients with shorter disease. Open symbols: HLA-B27-positive patients, filled symbols: HLA B27-negative patients. (with permission of *Arthritis & Rheumatism*, see ref. # 3)

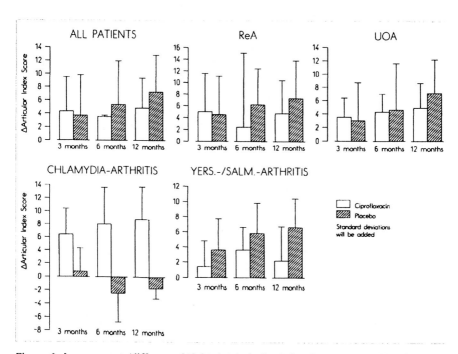

Figure 6. Improvement (difference [Δ] in the Articular Index Score among all patients and among subgroups of patients with reactive arthritis (ReA), undifferentiated oligoarthritis (UOA), *Chlamydia*-induced arthritis, and enteric arthritis (*Yersinia*-induced [Yers.] and *Salmonella*-induced [Salm.]) treated with ciprofloxacin or placebo at different time points. Values are the mean and SD. (with permission of *Arthritis & Rheumatism*, see ref. # 4)

placebo. We could not see any difference between the verum and the placebo group. The only difference we could see after three months was indeed in the group of patients with Chlamydia-induced arthritis in comparison to patients with arthritis after enteric infections (Figures 5, 6). We chose Ciprofloxacin although it is known to be not the best antibiotic for *C. trachomatis*, because we thought that enterobacteria might be more important and we wanted to have an antibiotic which would be effective against enterobacteria and at least partly effective against *C. trachomatis*. After a follow-up of 12 months we also saw an effect in the Ciprofloxacin group compared to the placebo group in patients with Chlamydia-induced arthritis (Figures 6, 7). Although the number of patients with a Chlamydia-induced arthritis was relatively small, we think that antibiotics might be effective. Another study has been done a while ago with tetracyclines which also showed an effect in the patients treated with antibiotics. But this older study also treated a relatively small group of patients with Chlamydia-induced arthritis.

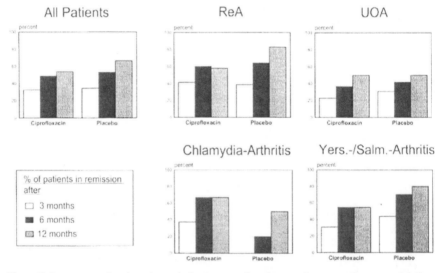

Figure 7. Percentage of patients in remission among all patients and among subgroups of patients with reactive arthritis (ReA), undifferentiated oligoarthritis (UOA), *Chlamydia*-induced arthritis, and enteric arthritis (*Yersinia*-induced [Yers.] and *Salmonella*-induced [Salm.]) treated with ciprofloxacin or placebo after 3 months (end of treatment), 6 months (first follow-up), and 12 months (second follow-up). (with permission of *Arthritis & Rheumatism*, see ref. # 4)

I was glad to learn earlier today from Dr. Saikku's data that also some positive effect was observed in the prevention of heart attacks in patients treated with Ciprofloxacin, because we are well aware that Ciprofloxacin might be not the best antibiotic for *C. trachomatis*.

In conclusion, *C. trachomatis* is a frequent cause of arthritis, while *C. pneumoniae* is a rather rare cause of arthritis. An inhibited TH1 response (locally and systemically) can be found in patients with reactive arthritis which might contribute to bacterial persistence *in vivo*.

Antibiotic treatment seems to be partly effective, although there is a study from Philadelphia reporting that there was no change either in the clinical course or in the detection of Chlamydia by PCR before and after treatment with antibiotics in 2 patients. We certainly need more and better studies about this. Because I think there might be a partly ineffective immune response, it must also be considered that, in addition to antibiotics, an additional stimulation of the immune system might be necessary to get rid of the bacteria which are difficult to attack.

References

1. Braun J, Laitko S, Treharne J, Eggens U, Wu P, Distler A, Sieper J (1994) *Chlamydia pneumoniae* – a new causative agent of reactive arthritis and undifferentiated oligoarthritis. Ann Rheum Dis 53: 100–105
2. Braun J, Tuszewski M, Eggens U, Mertz A, Schauer-Petrowskaja C, Döring E, Laitko S, Distler A, Sieper J, Ehlers S (1997) Use of nested PCR strategy simultaneously targeting DNA sequences of multiple bacterial species in inflammatory joint diseases. I. Screening of synovial fluid samples of patients with spondyloarthropathies and other arthritides. J Rheumatol 24: 1092–1100
3. Braun J, Yin Z, Spiller I, Siegert S, Rudwaleit M, Liu L, Radbruch A, Sieper J (1999) Low secretion of tumor necrosis factor A, but no other TH1 or TH2 cytokines, by peripheral blood mononuclear cells correlates with chronicity in reactive arthritis. Arthritis Rheum 42: 2039–2044
4. Sieper J, Fendler C, Laitko S, Sörensen H, Gripenberg-Lerche C, Hiepe F, Alten R, Keitel W, Groh A, Uksila J, Eggens U, Granfors K, Braun J (1999) No benefit of long-term ciprofloxacin treatment in patients with reactive arthritis and undifferentiated oligoarthritis: a three-month, multicenter, double-blind, randomized, placebo-controlled study. Arthritis Rheum 42: 1386–1396
5. Simon K, Seipelt E, Sieper J (1994) Divergent T cell cytokine patterns in arthritis. Proc Natl Acad Sci (USA) 91: 8562–8566
6. Wilkinson NZ, Kingsley G, Sieper J, Braun J, Ward ME (1998) Lack of correlation between the detection of *Chlamydia trachomatis* DNA in synovial fluid from patients with a range of rheumatic diseases and the presence of an antichlamydial immune response. Arthritis Rheum 41: 845–854
7. Yin J, Braun J, Neure L, Wu P, Liu L, Eggens U, Sieper J (1997) Crucial role of Interleukin-10/Interleukin-12 balance in the regulation of the type 2 T helper cytokine response in reactive arthritis. Arthritis Rheum 40: 1788–1797
8. Yin Z, Braun J, Neure L, Wu P, Eggens U, Krause A, Kamradt T, Sieper J (1997) T cell cytokine pattern in the joints of lyme arthritis patients and its regulation by cytokines and anticytokines. Arthritis Rheum 40: 69–79
9. Yin Z, Siegert S, Neure L, Grolms M, Liu L, Eggens U, Radbruch A, Braun J, Sieper J (1999) The elevated ratio of IFN-gamma/IL-4-positive T cells found in synovial fluid and synovial membrane of rheumatoid arthritis patients can be changed by IL-4 but not by IL-10 or TGFβ. Rheumatology 38: 1058–1067

Discussion

Hammerschlag:

For the treatment of *C. trachomatis* in urethritis with ciprofloxacin the efficacy rate of 50 % is far below what is considered to be acceptable, which has to be way over 90 %. The only antibiotic that might have a *C. trachomatis* indication actually is ofloxacin in multiple dose where it is about equivalent to doxycycline or anything else. Even going back to the Mayo study: only 8 patients got chinolones in this study, and the authors did not specify the duration of therapy but only dealt with dosing. The three chinolones, while they did not specify which patients actually got how many doses of, were ciprofloxacin or ofloxacin or others. We are talking about a very small number of patients, and I do not know what this really means.

Sieper:

I am not arguing that we should not use ciprofloxacin for *C. trachomatis*. But our results are encouraging to use an antibiotic which might be more effective than ciprofloxacin.

Anonymus:

Has anybody looked in connection with *C. pneumoniae* for cytokines?

Sieper:

Not that I am aware of.

Byrne:

Both Jim Summersgill and Charlotte Gaydos have data on the effects of INF-γ on *C. pneumoniae*, at least in people. It is similar to our experience with *C. trachomatis* where it is not eradicated but rather causes induction of a persistent state. On the other hand, in the rodent systems where inducible nitric oxide synthase seems to be the predominant activity induced by both IFN-γ and TNF-α, they do tend to eradicate.

3.5
Chlamydia pneumoniae, APOE genotype, and Alzheimer's disease

A.P. Hudson, H.C. Gérard, J.A. Whittum-Hudson, D.M. Appelt, B.J. Balin

Alzheimer's disease

Alzheimer's disease (AD) is a progressive neurodegenerative condition associated with atrophy and death of nerve cells in affected brain regions. This disease is relatively common, affecting 4 million or more individuals in the United States alone [1]. AD occurs in two relatively distinct forms: an early-onset, familial form and a more common late-onset, sporadic form. Incidence of the latter increases with increasing age, and AD is considered to be the most significant single cause of senile dementia. Indeed, a number of studies have indicated that at least half the total number of cases of dementia in the elderly are attributable to AD [2].

The specific etiology underlying the neuropathogenesis seen in virtually all AD patients is poorly understood. The *tau* protein is a normal cytoskeletal component, and evidence suggests that its deposition in neurofibrillary tangles (NFT) results from aberrant post-translational modifications of various types; deposition also may result from production of unusual forms of the protein itself *via* alternate splicing of the messenger encoding it [3–5]. It is not clear whether NFT are primary lesions in AD, or whether their formation is a response to other insults [6]. Neuritic senile plaques (NSP) are comprised of deposits of β-amyloid peptide (Aβ), and deposition of this peptide appears to be necessary for the neuronal degeneration characteristic of AD [7]. Aβ is derived from a region near the C-terminus of the amyloid precursor protein *via* protease digestion and is 39–42 amino acids long; encoded by the β*APP* gene on chromosome 21, the precise function(s) of amyloid precursor protein remain(s) unknown, although it is expressed in both neuronal and non-neuronal tissues [8].

In familial AD (FAD), mutations in the β*APP* gene are associated with increased Aβ deposition and the characteristic early and severe onset of symptoms [9]. Moreover, lesions in the unlinked genes encoding presenilin-1 (*PS-1*) and presenilin-2 (*PS-2*) have been shown to cause increased deposition of Aβ in FAD patients [*e.g.*, 10]. As with the β*APP* gene product, the precise function(s) of presenilin-1 and presenilin-2 remain unclear. Mutations in *PS-1* and *PS-2*, with those in β*APP*, appear to account for most FAD cases. However, the specific causes underlying NSP, as well as NFT, formation in late-onset AD remain to be established.

APOE allele types and Alzheimer's disease

The early-onset, FAD form of AD is primarily genetically-based, but late-onset AD, by far the most common form of the disease, is not [11]. One established risk factor for the latter is possession of the ε4 allele type of the *APOE* locus [7,12]. Not all patients with one or two ε4 alleles will ultimately develop AD, but presence of this allele type appears to increase risk for development of the disease several-fold [12]. Possession of ε4 is associated also with earlier onset and more rapid progression of the neurodegenerative process. However, a recent study suggested that ε4 alone is not a straightforward risk factor for AD, but rather that its product, in combination with infection by HSV-1, constitutes a risk factor [13]. This latter suggestion is consistent with observations concerning *C. pneumoniae* infection described below.

The *APOE* gene product itself is a serum apolipoprotein which performs a number of important functions, including several critical to the general homeostasis of plasma lipoproteins. In the nervous system, the three major ApoE protein isoforms (E2, E3, E4) are synthesized and secreted by astrocytes and macrophages [14]. In the heart, mRNA from the *APOE* gene is expressed by macrophages. The precise means by which the ε4 type gene product initiates, promotes, or maintains the neuropathogenesis process ending in AD remains to be elucidated, although some studies suggest that this gene product influences deposition of Aβ. ApoE4 does not appear to modulate expression of β*APP* or *PS-1* [15]; however, it has been reported to bind to Aβ with higher affinity than do the *APOE* ε2 and ε3 gene products in *in vitro* assays [16]. The ε4 gene product also has been reported to be present in NSP.

Pathogenesis and epidemiology of *Chlamydia pneumoniae*

Each of the four species comprising the Genus *Chlamydia* is pathogenic, and each is an obligate intracellular parasite of eukaryotic cells. Acquisition of *Chlamydia* species is *via* mucosal surfaces; *Chlamydia pneumoniae* is a respiratory pathogen, and thus its initial sites of infection are the oral and nasal mucosa [17]. This organism is a significant agent in acute respiratory infections, including pneumonia and bronchitis [17, 18]. Further, some recent studies have implicated *C. pneumoniae* in more severe pulmonary pathologies, including chronic obstructive pulmonary disease [19]. Infection with *C. pneumoniae* has been implicated in unexpected (non-respiratory) clinical manifestations, including arthritis [20] and atherosclerosis [21]. In the case of the latter, the bacterium has been identified in atheromatous plaques [22]; a high level of correlation exists between anti-*C. pneumoniae* antibody (Ab) titers and coronary artery disease. Importantly, recent *in vitro* studies suggest that *C. pneumoniae* infection induces foam cell formation and accumulation of cholesteryl esters within host cells under some conditions [23], thus providing direct biochemical evidence of a role for the organism in atherogenesis.

Epidemiologic studies from many sources indicate that *C. pneumoniae* is ubiquitous. Overall prevalence of infection with this organism is high in virtually all populations so far studied, and that prevalence appears to increase with increasing age [17, 18, 24]. That is, in areas where population densities are relatively low, children younger than 5–10 years of age rarely show anti-*C. pneumoniae* Ab, but incidence rises sharply after that age. In one study, for example, males 60 years and older showed a prevalence rate of 70 % [17, 24]. In more crowded regions, childhood infection with *C. pneumoniae* appears to be more common [17, 24]. A study from Scandinavia indicated that epidemics of *C. pneumoniae* occur every 5-7 yr, each lasting for a considerable period, and that most individuals incur several infections over a lifetime [17, 18, 24].

Chlamydia pneumoniae DNA in the Alzheimer's brain

Inflammation is a hallmark of sites of chlamydial infection, and it is also common in regions of neuropathology in the AD brain [25, 26]. Moreover, *C. pneumoniae* is ubiquitous in older adults, the susceptible population for late-onset AD. For these and a number of other reasons, we investigated whether there might be some association between *C. pneumoniae* infection and late-onset AD. We developed highly specific and sensitive PCR assays targeting chromosomal DNA sequences of *C. pneumoniae* [20], and we used them to assess DNA preparations from brain tissue samples from 19 AD, and an equal number of non-AD control, patients. Extensive positive and negative controls were included in each PCR screening assay run in these studies. As described in our initial publication [27], samples from brain regions showing characteristic neuropathology were PCR-positive for the organism in 17/19 AD patients; samples from cerebellum, a region usually less affected, from those AD patients were positive in four cases, and each of these four exhibited severe neuropathology in standard microscopic analysis. The two AD patient samples PCR-negative for *C. pneumoniae* exhibited less severe neuropathology in similar microscopic analyses. In contrast to results from AD patients, only one sample from an age-matched, non-AD control patient was positive in these screening assays, and that sample was only weakly positive [27].

In our original study, three control (non-AD) brain tissue samples assessed by PCR for *C. pneumoniae* DNA were derived from patients with multiple sclerosis (MS) [27]; in contrast to results from another recent study [28], all samples from each MS patient were PCR-negative for the organism in our assays. Since publication, we have extended control PCR screening assays to include brain tissue samples from patients with Parkinson's disease (PD), in order to determine whether the organism is present in the CNS in that context. In this new patient group, DNA samples prepared from temporal cortex and hippocampus were assayed from three non-AD/non-PD control individuals, three patients with PD, and two patients with *both* PD and AD. In PCR assays targeting the *C. pneumoniae* 16S rRNA gene, each sample from normal patients was negative, as were all samples from the PD patients; however, samples from each of the two patients with both PD and AD were PCR-positive for *C. pneumoniae* DNA (Figure 1); all patient samples were PCR-negative for *C. trachomatis* DNA in separate assays. Thus, both published data and those from recent unpublished studies indicate that DNA from *C. pneumoniae* is found in the AD brain, but it is rare in samples from congruent regions of control brains, including those from individuals with neurodegenerative diseases other than AD.

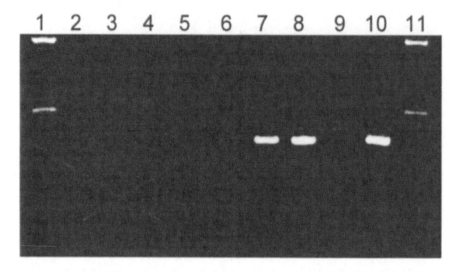

Figure 1. PCR assays targeting the *C. pneumoniae* 16S rRNA gene in nucleic acid samples from temporal cortex of seven patients. Preparation of DNA from brain tissues and PCR assays were as described in ref. [27]. Lanes are: 1, 100 bp size stds; PCR of DNA from 2, normal patient 1; 3, normal patient 2; 4, normal patient 3; 5, PD patient 1; 6, PD patient 2; 7, PD+AD patient 1; 8, PD+AD patient 2; 9, negative control (water only); 10, positive control (DNA from TW-183 EB); 11, 100 bp size stds.

Ultrastructural analysis of *Chlamydia pneumoniae* in the Alzheimer's brain

To confirm the PCR results and to visualize the organism in the AD brain, we used electron and immunoelectron microscopy (EM, IEM) to analyze brain tissue sections from AD and control patients. EM analyses revealed that areas of the hippocampus, temporal cortex, and/or other regions of AD brains displaying characteristic neuropathology contained objects that resembled chlamydial inclusions (Figure 2A), and within them structures whose morphology and size were consistent with those of the elementary and reticulate body (EB, RB) forms of the organism (Figures 2A, 2B). We also identified structures resembling RB in the process of cell division (not shown), suggesting that the organisms represented vegetatively growing chlamydia. We could identify no similar structures in non-AD control brains in parallel analyses (*e.g.*, Figure 2C). For IEM, we used a commercial monoclonal Ab (mAb) targeting an outer membrane protein (OMP) of *C. pneumoniae*, and this mAb clearly identified the objects resembling chlamydial EB and RB as authentic *C. pneumoniae*. Labeling not tightly associated with positive cells was always rare in the AD patients analyzed by IEM, and examination of stained sections from the PCR-negative patients showed no significant or specific labeling. Thus, both EM and IEM studies of affected brain regions of AD patients confirmed that *C. pneumoniae* is present in those tissues. (See [27] for extensive controls and discussion.)

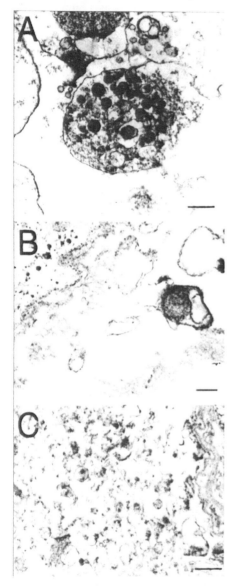

Figure 2. EM analyses of AD brains revealed apparent cytoplasmic vesicles, EB, and RB of *C. pneumoniae*. **Panel A**, typical chlamydia-like vesicle containing apparent EB and RB from temporal cortex of an AD patient. **Panel B**, classic pear-shaped form of *C. pneumoniae* EB in temporal cortex of an AD patient. **Panel C**, control brain tissues showed no similar structures. Bars=0.5 μm (*A*), 0.25 μm (*B*), 1.0 μm (*C*).

Culture of *Chlamydia pneumoniae* from Alzheimer's brain tissue

To provide additional confirmation that *C. pneumoniae* was indeed present in AD brain tissues, we cultured the organism from homogenates of AD and control samples, using the human monocyte cell line THP-1 as host. Immunocytochemistry using the anti-OMP mAb was performed on cytospun THP-1 cells after culture with brain homogenates. THP-1 cells incubated with homogenates from temporal cortex of control brains were negative for *C. pneumoniae* using the anti-OMP mAb. In contrast, THP-1 cells from cultures incubated with homogenates from temporal cortex of AD patient samples displayed strong immunopositivity using the mAb after one passage (72 hr) and after two passages (7 d). We further visualized *C. pneumoniae* inclusions within infected THP-1 cells by transmission EM; these studies clearly demonstrated the organism after both passages. Thus, infectious *C. pneumoniae* were present in brain tissue from the AD patients subjected to culture analysis, but the organism was absent in congruent tissues from non-AD patients studied [27].

Immunohistochemical analyses

Immunostaining of tissues from affected regions of AD brains and congruent regions from non-AD brains employed two mAb, a genus-specific mAb targeting the lipopolysaccharide (LPS) of *Chlamydia*, and the species-specific anti-OMP mAb employed in IEM studies. In sections from several AD brains, we found staining in perivascular regions of blood vessels in the neuropil, and in microglia- and astroglia-like cells not adjacent to such vessels. In sections from non-AD patients, no significant labeling was seen using either mAb, and immunostaining of AD brains with an irrelevant mAb (anti-CD54) showed little background signal, confirming the specificity of positive reactions with the two *Chlamydia*-specific mAb. Thus, immunohistochemical analyses confirmed the presence of *C. pneumoniae* in affected AD brain regions, and importantly, those analyses localized the bacterium to non-neuronal, resident central nervous system cells [27].

We identified the cell types harboring *C. pneumoniae* in the brain *via* double immunolabeling. Double labeling of sections from AD brains using the anti-chlamydial LPS mAb and an anti-glial fibrillary acidic protein (GFAP) mAb showed that astroglia function as host cells for *C. pneumoniae* in the AD brain. Similar studies using an anti-iNOS Ab in combination with the anti-OMP mAb identified activated microglia as hosts. The chlamydia-infected cells surrounding blood vessels in the AD brain are pericytes, since they labeled with the anti-iNOS and anti-OMP Ab (see [27]). These cells also express the CD68 surface marker, and double immunolabeling studies using a mAb targeting this protein, with the anti-OMP mAb, confirmed that these hosts are pericytes. The level of autofluorescence given by tissue sections in all staining experiments was extremely low. Thus, at least three cell types, astroglia, microglia, and pericytes, harbor *C. pneumoniae* in the AD brain. This diversity of cell types infected with the organism in the AD brain may explain in part the complexity of the pathogenesis process.

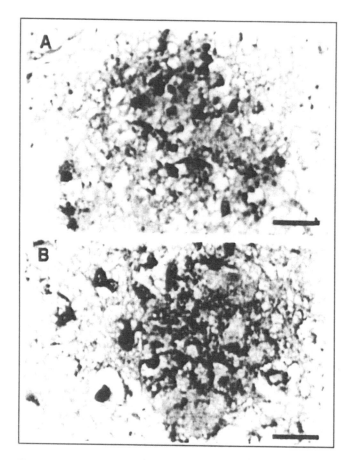

Figure 3. *C. pneumoniae*-infected host cells are located in the immediate vicinity of PHF-*tau* protein deposition in neurites within NFT. **Panel A**, section from hippocampus of an AD patient labeled with the PHF-1 mAb; **Panel B**, a consecutive section from the same series labeled with the anti-*C. pneumoniae* OMP mAb. Bars = 100 μm.

The PHF-1 mAb identifies neuritic pathology in AD brain tissues. Staining of consecutive tissue sections from AD brains with the PHF-1 and anti-OMP mAb, respectively, demonstrated the presence of chlamydia-infected glial cells near PHF-*tau* protein deposition in neurites in each of the several AD patients so analyzed (Figure 3A, 3B). For the same AD patients, similarly performed immunolabeling of brain areas with little or no neuropathology showed that essentially no cells harboring *C. pneumoniae* were present; no infected cells were identified in any non-AD brain examined [27]. Thus, chlamydia-infected astroglia and microglia in the AD brain are concentrated in regions of characteristic neuropathology.

Chlamydia pneumoniae infection and *APOE* allele types

We reasoned that if the *APOE* ε4 allele type (or its gene product) is associated with development of AD [12], and if *C. pneumoniae* is associated with the same disease, then some relationship might exist between ε4 and the bacterium. To address this question, we asked whether any relationship could be demonstrated between *APOE* genotype and synovial infection with *C. pneumoniae*, since DNA from the organism has been identified in synovial tissue from some arthritis patients [20]. Nucleic acids from synovial tissue of a large patient group (average age 43 yr) were screened by PCR for DNA from *C. trachomatis*, *C. pneumoniae*, and other bacteria, the latter using a "pan-bacteria" primer set. *APOE* genotype was defined by a standard PCR-based method for all patients in each of four resulting groups comprised of about 35 individuals each: positive for *C. trachomatis* only, *C. pneumoniae* only, other bacteria only, or no bacteria. RT-PCR was used to assess synovial *APOE* expression, and these assays confirmed *APOE* mRNA in synovial tissue. Determination of *APOE* genotype showed that patients PCR-negative in all assays, and those positive only in the *C. trachomatis*- and pan-bacteria- (excludes *Chlamydia*) directed assays, showed distributions of the ε2, ε3, and ε4 alleles which closely mirrored those of the general population ([29]; Table 1). In sharp contrast, 68 % of patients with *C. pneumoniae* DNA in synovium had a copy of ε4 [30]. As developed in the following section, we suspect that this observation indicates a role for the ε4 gene product in promotion of infectivity, dissemination, or some other aspect of the pathobiology of the organism, in turn significantly strengthening the apparent association between infection with *C. pneumoniae* and development of late-onset AD.

Table 1. Distribution of *ApoE* genotypes in four patient study groups.

Study groups	*APOE* genotypes (as percent of group total)[a]					
	ε2/ε2	ε2/ε3	ε2/ε4	ε3/ε3	ε3/ε4	ε4/ε4
C. trachomatis	0	4 %	0	83 %	13 %	0
C. pneumoniae[b]	0	9 %	12 %	23 %	56 %	0
Pan Bacteria	0	13 %	0	70 %	17 %	0
No Bacteria	3 %	18 %	3 %	56 %	20 %	0

[a] normal population frequency for each allele is: ε2=7.5 %, ε3=78.6 %, ε4=13.5 %, ε1+ε5=0.4 % [ref. 29]
[b] group includes six patients PCR-positive for both *C. trachomatis* and *C. pneumoniae*

Future research directions

Neurologic diseases can be caused by bacteria and viruses, and even infection with agents that do not directly target the nervous system can elicit neuropathologic side-effects [31]. Some bacteria associated with neurologic disease are intracellular pathogens with the ability to inhibit phagosome-lysosome fusion and to attach to, penetrate, and survive in a long-term manner within host cells. Our current understanding of *Chlamydia pneumoniae* is congruent with many aspects of other studies of bacterial infection in diverse neurological conditions. A number of earlier studies attempted to define an etiologic relationship between infection with various viruses or bacterial species and the development of AD, but no such link has been clearly demonstrated as yet [32, 33]. As mentioned earlier, one group identified HSV-1 infection as a risk factor for development of AD in individuals either heterozygous or homozygous for the *APOE* ε4 allele [13]. In addition to viruses and bacteria, prions have been considered in the pathogenesis of AD and discarded [34], and no clear evidence has been forthcoming concerning the possible roles of environmental factors, including diet and exposure to aluminum [1]. One recent study suggested that head trauma may be associated with Aβ deposition in individuals carrying *APOE* ε4 [35].

The data summarized here regarding the presence and location of *C. pneumoniae* in the brain appear to be the first to demonstrate relatively consistent proximity of a known bacterial pathogen to regions of standard AD-related neuropathology. It is of interest that we identified the organism only in AD brain materials, but not in congruent brain samples from patients with MS or PD, or in samples from patients without neurologic disease; the numbers of samples assayed from patients with MS and PD was, however, extremely small, and more study of the presence of *C. pneumoniae* in brain tissues from patients with various neurodegenerative diseases is required. Without question, it will also be important for other laboratories to replicate our PCR, immunohistochemistry, EM, IEM, and culture observations in larger AD and control patient populations.

Regardless, the initial demonstration of a known bacterial pathogen in close and apparently exclusive conjunction with the neuropathologic structures characteristic of AD offers a tempting opportunity for speculation concerning possible mechanisms of pathogenesis in this disease. We do not, of course, know at what point in time and under what physiologic conditions *C. pneumoniae* reaches the central nervous system in susceptible individuals. It seems unlikely, however, that it does so simply as a result of normal aging processes, since only a small proportion of brain samples from our age-matched non-AD control patients was PCR-positive for DNA from the organism. Moreover, the organism does not appear to be present in brain tissues from individuals with neurodegenerative diseases other than AD.

C. pneumoniae has been identified in circulating mononuclear cells [*e.g.*, 36], and it seems reasonable to suspect that this vehicle might be one means of transport for the organism from respiratory mucosa to the brain. In preliminary studies, we investigated another route by which the bacterium might reach the brain. Distribution of NSP/NFT vary among affected areas of the AD brain and among individuals with the disease, but one region always affected is the hippocampus; this structure is in close proximity to the olfactory bulb, suggesting to us that the bacterium might reach the hippocampus from that structure *via* passage from the nasal mucosa through the olfactory nerve tract. The olfactory bulb is not normally obtained during autopsy at our institutions, but we procured it from two AD patients and screened for *C. pneumoniae* DNA by the same PCR assays used in our initial studies. Both olfactory bulbs were PCR-positive for the organism, and RT-PCR showed that mRNA from *C. pneumoniae* was present in that structure (Figure 4), suggesting that the bacterium was viable and metabolically active in those samples. We do not know from this very preliminary observation whether the direction of spread of infection is from olfactory bulb to hippocampus or *vice versa*, nor do we know, if spread occurs by the former route, whether this is a primary or secondary means for *C. pneumoniae* to access the central nervous system. In either case, the question of how this organism reaches the brain across the blood–brain barrier must be a major focus of future research.

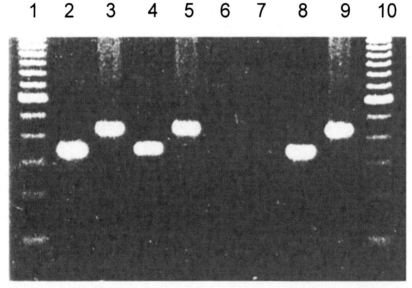

Figure 4. RT-PCR analyses demonstrating *C. pneumoniae* messengers in total RNA prepared from olfactory bulbs taken from 2 AD patients. Lanes are: 1, 100 bp size standards; 2, *ompA*-directed assay using RNA from an AD patient; 3, 16S rRNA-directed assay using RNA from the same AD patient; 4, *ompA*-directed assay using RNA from a second AD patient; 5, 16S rRNA-directed assay using RNA from the second patient; 6, negative control (no nucleic acids added) for *ompA* assay; 7, negative control (no nucleic acids added) for 16S-directed assay; 8, positive control for *ompA* assay; 9, positive control for 16S assay. Both positive control assays used chromosomal DNA from *C. pneumoniae* (strain TW-183).

Data from a number of studies indicate that treatment of AD patients with non-steroidal anti-inflammatory drugs (NSAIDS) has beneficial effects on those individuals [37]. These drugs are known to inhibit cyclo-oxygenases, which may block to some extent the calcium-dependent post-synaptic cascade that induces excitotoxic cell death in NMDA-reactive neurons in AD. The observation that NSAIDS are useful in treating AD clearly suggests that the inflammatory process characteristic of the AD brain is an important component of neuropathogenesis. Current opinion holds that such inflammation results primarily from deposition of Aβ in NSP [38]. However, it seems probable that at least some portion of the inflammation associated with the AD brain would be attributable to chlamydial infection, once infection of astrocytes, microglia, and pericytes within the brain has been established. Thus, more studies of NSAID use, perhaps in combination with antibiotic regimens, may prove to be useful therapeutically for AD patients.

Our observations regarding the presence of *C. pneumoniae* in the AD brain do not demonstrate a causal relationship between infection with the organism and this disease. As indicated just above, however, they do suggest some relationship between *C. pneumoniae* and several aspects of AD-related neuropathology. We contend that this suggestion is strengthened significantly by our demonstration of an association between *C. pneumoniae* and the *APOE* ε4 allele type. The function of E4 type apolipoprotein in synovial infection by *C. pneumoniae* is unknown, of course, as is its role in promoting development of late-onset AD. We strongly suspect, however, that the association between synovial *C. pneumoniae* and possession of ε4 is simply another aspect of the relationship between AD and this allele. That is, we contend that the extremely high proportion of *C. pneumoniae*-infected arthritis patients possessing ε4 indicates that this gene product somehow promotes one or more as yet unknown aspects of the pathobiology of *C. pneumoniae*. In turn, this suggests that brain infection by the organism in individuals possessing ε4 would result from the same mechanism as does synovial infection with the organism [30]. These arguments further indicate that possession of ε4 may be only a surrogate marker for risk of development of late-onset AD, but a direct risk factor for infection with, or disease from, *C. pneumoniae*. It will be of much interest to define the role of the *APOE* ε4 gene product on the pathobiology of *C. pneumoniae*, an issue now under vigorous investigation by this group.

A number of other critical issues must be addressed in relation to the potential role of *C. pneumoniae* in the pathogenesis of late-onset AD. First, it will be important to determine whether the organism infecting AD brain tissues represents a specific neurotropic strain. We have begun this determination, and data available thus far suggest that the bacteria identified in our earlier studies are variable, at least in terms of the DNA sequence of the *ompA* gene. Another critical question concerns the detailed effects of *C. pneumoniae* infection on astrocytes and microglia, specifically in terms of modulation of amyloid precursor protein production and/or modification, *tau* modification, *etc*. Such studies should provide relatively direct evidence as to whether *C. pneumoniae* plays an overt role in the neuropathogenesis ending in AD.

References

1. Keefover RW (1996) The clinical epidemiology of Alzheimer's disease. Neurol Clin 14: 337–351
2. Evans DA, Funkenstein HH, Albert MS, et al. (1989) Prevalence of Alzheimer's disease in a community population of older persons. JAMA 262: 2551–2556
3. Lee VM-Y, Balin BJ, Otvos L, Trojanowski JQ (1991) A68 – a major subunit of paired helical filaments and derivatized forms of normal tau. Science 251: 675–679

4. Alonso A, Grundke-Iqbal I, Iqbal K (1996) Alzheimer's disease hyperphosphorylated tau sequesters normal tau into tangles of filaments and disassembles microtubules. Nature Med 2: 783–787
5. Wang J-Z, Grundke-Iqbal I, Iqbal K (1996) Glycosylation of microtubule-associated protein tau: an abnormal post-translational modification in Alzheimer's disease. Nature Med 2: 871–875
6. Goedert M (1993) Tau protein and the neurofibrillary pathology of Alzheimer's disease. Trends Neurosci 16: 460–465
7. Schellenberg GD (1995) Genetic dissection of Alzheimer's disease, a heterogeneous disorder. Proc Natl Acad Sci (USA) 92: 8552–8559
8. Selkoe DJ, Podlisny MD, et al. (1988) β-amyloid precursor protein of AD occurs at 110- to 135-kilodalton membrane-associated proteins in neural and nonneural tissues. Proc Natl Acad Sci (USA) 85: 7341–7345
9. Yankner BA (1996) New clues to Alzheimer's disease: unraveling the roles of amyloid and tau. Nature Med 2: 850–852
10. Scheuner D, Eckman C, Jensen M, et al. (1996) Secreted amyloid β-protein similar to that in the senile plaques of AD is increased *in vivo* by the presenilin 1 and 2 mutations linked to familial AD. Nature Med 2: 864–870
11. Ray WJ, Ashall F, Goate AM (1998) Molecular pathogenesis of sporadic and familial forms of Alzheimer's disease. Mol Med Today 4: 151–157
12. Roses AD (1996) Apolipoprotein E alleles as risk factor in Alzheimer's disease. Annu Rev Med 47: 387–400
13. Itzhaki RJ, Lin WR, Shang D, et al. (1997) Herpes simplex virus type 1 in brain and risk of Alzheimer's disease. Lancet 349: 241–244
14. Boyles JK, Pitas RE, Wilson E, et al. (1985) ApoE associated with astrocytic glia of the central nervous system and with nonmyelinating glia of the peripheral nervous system. J Clin Invest 76: 1501–1513
15. Haan J, Van Broeckhoven C, van Duijn CM, et al. (1994) The apolipoprotein E ε4 allele does not influence the clinical expression of the amyloid precursor protein gene codon 693 or 692 mutations. Ann Neurol 36: 434–437
16. Strittmatter WJ, Weisgraber KH, Huang DY, et al. (1993) Binding of human apolipoprotein E to synthetic amyloid β peptide: isoform-specific effects and implications for late-onset Alzheimer's disease; essentially all Alzheimer's patients also show a severe deficit in cholinergic nerve function Alzheimer disease. Proc Natl Acad Sci (USA) 90: 8098–8102
17. Grayston JT (1992) *Chlamydia pneumoniae*, strain TWAR pneumonia. Annu Rev Med 43: 317–323
18. Grayston JT, Campbell LA, Kuo CC, et al. (1990) A new respiratory tract pathogen: *Chlamydia pneumoniae* strain TWAR. J Infect Dis 161: 618–625
19. Von Hertzen LC (1998) *Chlamydia pneumoniae* and its role in chronic obstructive pulmonary disease. Ann Med 30: 27–37
20. Schumacher HR, Gérard HC, Arayssi T, et al. (1999). Lower prevalence of *Chlamydia pneumoniae* DNA compared with *Chlamydia trachomatis* DNA in synovial tissue of arthritis patients. Arthritis Rheum 42:1889–1893
21. Kuo CC, Grayston JT, Campbell LA, et al. (1995) *Chlamydia pneumoniae* (TWAR) in coronary arteries of young adults (15–34 years old). Proc Natl Acad Sci (USA) 92: 6911–6914

22. Campbell LA, O'Brien ER, Cappuccio AL, et al. (1995) Detection of *Chlamydia pneumoniae* TWAR in human coronary atherectomy tissues. J Infect Dis 172: 585–588
23. Kalayoglu MV, Byrne GI (1998) Induction of macrophage foam cell formation by *Chlamydia pneumoniae*. J Infect Dis 177: 725–729
24. Leinonen M (1993) Pathogenetic mechanisms and epidemiology *of Chlamydia pneumoniae*. Eur Heart J 14: 57–61
25. Ward ME (1995) The immunobiology and immunopathology of chlamydial infections. APMIS 103: 769–796
26. Chen S, Frederickson RC, Brunden KR (1996) Neuroglial-mediated immunoinflammatory responses in Alzheimer's disease: complement activation and therapeutic approaches. Neurobiol Aging 17: 781–787
27. Balin BJ, Gérard HC, Arking EJ, et al. (1998) Identification and localization of *Chlamydia pneumoniae* in the Alzheimer's brain. Med Microbiol Immunol 187: 23–42
28. Sriram S, Mitchell W, Stratton C (1998) Multiple sclerosis association with *Chlamydia pneumoniae* infection of the CNS. Neurology 50: 571–572
29. Ordovas JM, Litwack-Klein L, Wilson PWF, et al. (1987) ApoE isoform phenotyping methodology and population frequency with identification of apoE1 and apoE5. J Lipid Res 28: 371–380
30. Gérard HC, Wang GF, Balin BJ, et al. (1999) Frequency of apolipoprotein E (APOE) allele types in patients with Chlamydia-associated arthritis and other arthritides. Microb Pathog 26: 35–42
31. Bolton CF, Young GB, Zochodne DW (1993) The neurological consequences of sepsis. Ann Neurol 33: 94–100
32. Mann DM, Tinkler AM, Yates PO (1983) Neurological disease and herpes simplex virus. An immunohistochemical study. Acta Neurol 60: 24–28
33. Pogo BG, Casals J, Elizan TS (1987) A study of viral genomes and antigens in brains of patients with Alzheimer's disease. Brain 110: 907–915
34. Mathews WB (1986) Unconventional virus infection and neurological disease. Neuropath Appl Neurobiol 12: 111–116
35. Nicoll JAR, Roberts GW, Graham DI (1995) Apolipoprotein E ε4 allele is associated with deposition of amyloid β-protein following head injury. Nature Med 1: 135–137
36. Moazed TC, Kuo CC, Patten DL, et al. (1996) Experimental rabbit models *of Chlamydia pneumoniae* infection. Am J Pathol 148: 667–676
37. Breitner JC (1996) The role of anti-inflammatory drugs in the prevention and treatment of Alzheimer's disease. Annu Rev Med 47: 401–411
38. Lue L-H, Brachova L, Civin WH, Rogers J (1996) Inflammation, Aβ deposition, and neurofibrillary tangle formation as correlates of Alzheimer's disease neurodegeneration. J Neuropathol Exp Neurol 55: 1083–1088

Discussion

Straube:

Are the amplification products in PCR in Alzheimer patients the same as in the positive control with *C. pneumoniae*, or are they different in size?

Hudson:
They are the same size. That is, the size of the PCR products we obtained was what we expected. One of the assays was the Gaydos assay, targeting 16S rRNA gene. We got precisely the right size product and, in fact, confirmed this product in the initial study by hybridization with an internal probe. We have since cloned out a number of those PCR products and sequenced them, and they are from *C. pneumoniae* without question. We also have an *ompA*-directed assay that we used routinely, as reported in the paper, and other assays targeting the molecular weight 60,000 heat-shock protein and the KDO transferase that was published a number of years ago. We have sequenced some of each of these products, and they are what we think they are.

Byrne:
A question regarding *APOE* ε4, is it actually part of the LDL that interacts with the receptor?

Hudson:
My understanding is that it is not. I am not an *APOE* or a lipoprotein expert, but my understanding is that ApoE lipoprotein is the primary lipoprotein generated in the nervous system. It is made elsewhere as well, as we showed in synovial tissue. The general function of ApoE lipoprotein has to do with homeostasis of other lipoproteins in the blood stream and elsewhere. But its precise functions in terms of LDL I just don't know. I am sure somebody does.

Byrne:
I am wondering whether there is some sort of unique receptor situation associated with that particular allele of *APOE*. Perhaps we are talking about having cells that are more susceptible to take the Chlamydia up.

Hudson:
Yes, it could be infectivity, or it could be survivability in the monocytes that transport it around and deposit it in vessels, in brain etc. We actually are taking a look at this now, but we don't have any data to give as yet.

Byrne:
I am also interested in the fact that you seem to have great strain variability, especially in the *ompA* gene, and I guess that would not be what others experience.

Hudson:
They all look like AR39, but none are identical to AR39. We were surprised at this variability also, and that is why we are sequencing two or three clones from each of the patient samples. It is a lot of sequencing to do, but we want to make sure that we are not looking at a reading mistake by the *Taq* polymerase. In fact, we started sequence analysis using a kind of *Taq* polymerase with high fidelity, and we saw differences. We immediately went to a second clone or third clone from that same region from each of the same patients, and then looked in other

patients as well. Every sequence difference that we have seen has been confirmed in other clones. I don't know why we are seeing so much variability. We are not seeing 50 changes per strain or per patient sample, but two changes, one change, three changes. Even that is a bit more than we expected. I don't know why that is the case.

Brade:
I think *C. pneumoniae* is much more heterogeneous than one has the impression of from looking in the literature, where people have tried to make it one microorganism, nearly clonally expanded. I think that is for simple patent reasons.

Hudson:
Yes, right.

Brade:
One should not forget that TW-183 does not come from the lung but was isolated from a trachoma case, and IOL207, too. The koala strain is a *C. pneumoniae* strain. The N17 is a horse strain of *C. pneumoniae*. So obviously, *C. pneumoniae* is very heterogeneous, and I am not surprised to see different biovars which you cannot analyze with the tools we have at present. Even if you would sequence the whole genome of these strains, a single amino acid change can make the difference as to whether it is of this or that biotype.

Byrne:
But the non-human strains even have a plasmid, and there are a lot of differences there. As far as I know, human *C. pneumoniae* isolates don't.

Brade:
But they are much closer to human *C. pneumoniae* than to any other chlamydial strain.

Byrne:
Again, it may be a unique form of Chlamydia, but I am not talking about biovar differences but about genetic differences. Just based on the sequence information we have, with the exception of what Alan just told us, I think this genetic homogeneity is based on sequences we know.

Brade:
Are the isolates you have still surviving upon repeated passages?

Hudson:
We have not yet grown them out from our freezer cultures. We initially grew them up at two passages, directly out of the brain homogenates from the two Alzheimer patients. The controls, of course, were negative. We immediately froze them down because we knew that sometimes the strains do not last very long in culture. We all actually froze them down immediately, rather than doing experi-

ments on them immediately, because I knew I was moving to Detroit, and that the other laboratories involved in this were all moving also. We did not want to have them going as we were moving. The intention is that, as soon as we get back, we will take these isolates out of the freezer, wake them up and see if they will grow. That is why we have not done anything to date.

Stille:
As simple clinicians we have to state that Alzheimer's disease is a specialized brain amyloidosis. Do you have an opinion on the pathogenesis of the links between Chlamydia and brain amyloidosis? Do you have an idea who produces the amyloid which probably, in the end, brings the patients to dementia?

Hudson:
I have wondered whether this would come up. There is a good deal of data and a quite lively debate in the literature about this. The one situation that I know something about is Down's syndrome patients. These patients tend to develop dementia, and many of them die early of this dementia. So is there a relationship between the *APOE* allele type and people who have amyloid plaques in Down's syndrome? There is a debate in the literature saying that presence of $\epsilon 2$ appears to protect patients from this kind of problem, and that $\epsilon 4$ makes them more susceptible to this dementia due to plaques. We have not yet really looked at Down's syndrome patients. We have access to some samples, and we arranged just before we left that we would obtain and analyze them for *C. pneumoniae*. Amyloidosis may be a kind of general phenomenon. There was some relationship published in a paper about two years ago between amyloidosis and rheumatoid arthritis.

Stille:
This is classical amyloidosis.

Hudson:
Yes, that's right. There was some argument in that paper which I thought was pretty well done, but nobody has seemed to follow it up. We have some access to rheumatoid patients, and maybe we will take a look at those things.

Stille:
Maybe one clue observation is the so-called dementia pugilistica, the dementia of boxers and of the Alzheimer type. Certain boxers suffer from an early-onset Alzheimer's without genetic background, and maybe it has something to do with this, too.

Hudson:
This will be interesting to look at. I had not thought of this.

3.6
Association of *Chlamydia pneumoniae* with Multiple Sclerosis: Protocol for detection of *C. pneumoniae* in the CSF and summary of preliminary results

C.W. Stratton, S. Sriram, S. Yao, A. Tharp, L. Ding, J.D. Bannan, W.M. Mitchell

Introduction

We have reported a case of CNS infection with *C. pneumoniae* in a patient with rapidly progressive MS [27]. In this patient, *C. pneumoniae* was isolated from the CSF, and therapy with antimicrobial agents directed against this pathogen paralleled marked neurologic improvement. These observations prompted a prospective evaluation of the association of this organism with MS [26]. The purpose of this communication is to again summarize our findings and, more importantly, describe in detail the protocol in order that these optimized methods can be easily followed by others who wish to study the association of *C. pneumoniae* and MS.

Materials and methods

Patients and patient selection

Approval for entry to the study for both MS patients and other neurological diseases (OND) controls was obtained from the Institutional Review Board of Vanderbilt University School of Medicine. Patients were recruited for the study from the Multiple Sclerosis clinic at Vanderbilt Medical Center. Patients who satisfied the Poser criteria for the diagnosis of clinically definite MS were recruited for the study. These included 17 patients who, at the time of ascertainment, had clinically definite relapsing remitting MS and 20 patients who were in the progressive phase of the disease. Age- and gender-matched controls were recruited from OND control patients in whom CSF was being obtained for diagnostic studies.

Direct fluorescent antibody stain for C. pneumoniae *from CSF*

Although not described in either the case report [27] or the prospective study [26], we have also successfully used a direct fluorescent antibody (DFA) staining method to detect *C. pneumoniae* in the CSF. We include this DFA method for the sake of completeness. The procedure is done as follows: A large volume of CSF 5 ml is first centrifuged (Centra-8R; International Equipment Company [IEC], Needham, MA) at ambient temperature for 1 hour at 4,500 × gravity in order to concentrate any EBs. Next, EBs/cells in this concentrated CSF sample are directly deposited onto slides using a Cytospin 2 (Shandon Lipshow, Pittsburgh, PA). The Cytospin 2 uses centrifugal force to deposit a monolayer of bacteria or cells in a defined area on glass slides. Approximately 300 µl of the spun CSF sediment is then deposited in a single chamber Cytofunnel sample chamber with integral filter card and spun in the Cytospin 2 at 1000 × gravity for 10 minutes. The Cytospin slide is then fixed in cold acetone for 10 minutes and washed twice with PBS buffer, blocked with 1 % BSA – 0.15 % Tween 20 in PBS for 1 hour. The slide is finally stained with a *C. pneumoniae*-specific fluoresceine-conjugated mouse monoclonal antibody 1:50 dilution (Washington Research Foundation [WRF], Seattle, WA) at 37°C for 30 minutes. The stained slides are examined under epifluorescence using a Nikon Diaphot-TMD microscope (Nikon, Garden City, NY) with a B filter cassette.

Cell cultures of C. pneumoniae *from CSF*

Cell cultures of CSF are done using an optimized cell culture protocol for *C. pneumoniae* derived from published methods [2, 13, 16, 17, 21, 28, 29]. Strict quality control measures are considered essential in this method and include the following. All cell lines, fetal calf serum (FCS), media, and liquid reagents used in this optimized procedure are *Chlamydia*-free by PCR/Southern hybridization of concentrated samples. The PCR/Southern hybridization assay is included in the cell culture procedure as an on-going quality control measure. All manipulations of CSF samples and/or shell vials in which contamination might occur are performed in laminar-flow hoods (BL3) that are under continuous ultraviolet light when not in use.

In this optimized cell culture method, approximately 80,000 HL cells (WRF) are seeded in shell vials with 12 mm coverslips in order to obtain 85–90 % confluency by the day of inoculation. Before inoculation, cells are pretreated with diethylaminoethyl-dextran 30 mg/l (DEAE-Dextran; GIBCO BRL, Gaithersburg, MD) for 15 minutes, and rinsed 6 times in Hank's Balanced Salt Solution (HBSS; GIBCO).

At least 300 µl of a recently collected CSF sample is used for culture. However, the use of an increased volume of CSF will aid detection. To this CSF sample, 200 µl of trypsin (0.25 %) ethylenediaminetetraacetic acid (1 mM) EDTA (GIBCO) in HBSS (GIBCO) at pH 7.2 is added to achieve a final concentration of 0.1 % trypsin. Potential EBs in the CSF sample then are concentrated by centrifugation at ambient temperature for 45–60 minutes at 12,000 × gravity in a microcentrifuge; the resulting pellet is resuspended in 1 ml of plain Iscoves medium (GIBCO). This concentrated CSF sample provides an inoculum of 0.5 ml that is added to each of two shell vials and centrifuged at 4°C for 1 hour at 1,800 × gravity in a Sorvall RT6000 swinging bucket rotor.

For laboratories without the capability of providing 12,000 × gravity, an alternative method should be possible. This method would aspirate a large volume (2–4 ml) of the trypsin/EDTA-treated CSF through a 0.1 µm filter Super Acrodisc 25 syringe P/N S4651 (Gelman Sciences, Ann Arbor, MI) in order to concentrate potential chlamydial EBs. Potential EBs trapped by this filter could be collected by pushing 1 ml of the filtered CSF back through the filter. This backflow sample of CSF could then be used for the culture inoculum or for PCR analysis. It is essential that 0.1 μm maximal pore size or less be used since 0.2 μm pore size allows passage of EBs.

To the spun shell vials is added 0.5 ml of Iscoves (GIBCO) containing 20 % FCS (HyClone, Logan, UT), 4 mM L-glutamine (Sigma Chemicals, St. Louis, MO), 4 mg/l cyclohexamide, and 100 mg/l gentamicin (Sigma). The vials are then incubated at 35°C with 5 % CO_2 for 7 days with additional centrifugation 4°C for 1 hour at 1,800 × gravity on days 4, 5, and 6. Continuous propagation for 14 days is achieved by a single culture passage after 7 days followed by a second incubation period of 7 days.

For passage, each shell vial is sonicated for 15 seconds (Braun Sonic U, Allentown, PA) and centrifuged at ambient temperature for 10 minutes at low speed 600 × gravity to remove debris. The supernatant is centrifuged at ambient temperature for 45–60 minutes at 12,000 × gravity. This pellet is resuspended in 1 ml Iscoves (GIBCO) and 0.5 ml used to inoculate each of duplicate fresh DEAE-Dextran-treated cell monolayers. This passage culture is centrifuged at 4°C for 1 hour at 1,800 × gravity at the time of subculture as well as again on days 11, 12, and 13.

At the end of day 14, the cells on coverslips are fixed in cold acetone for 10 minutes and washed twice with PBS buffer, blocked with 1 % BSA – 0.15 % Tween 20 in PBS for 1 hour. The monolayers are then stained with a *C. pneumoniae*-specific fluoresceine-conjugated mouse monoclonal antibody 1:50 dilution (WRF) and Evan's blue 3 ml/l in PBS – 1 % BSA – 0.15 % Tween 20 at 37°C for 30 minutes. The stained coverslips are examined under epi-fluorescence using a Nikon Diaphot – TMD microscope (Nikon) with a B filter cassette. In the presence of Evan's blue counter-stain, the emission spectrum is shifted toward the infrared for this particular monoclonal antibody.

PCR detection of the MOMP gene of C. pneumoniae

The presence of *C. pneumoniae* in the CNS was evaluated by PCR methods similar to those published [3, 6, 20, 22]. All reagents used in this procedure should be demonstrated by PCR to be *Chlamydia*-free. All testing should include negative sterile distilled water as well as positive controls that progress through the entire PCR procedure. PCR DNA amplification of the *C. pneumoniae* MOMP gene from CSF specimens is done as follows: To at least 300 μl of CSF sample, 200 μl of trypsin (0.25 %) - EDTA 1 mM (GIBCO) in HBSS (GIBCO) at pH 7.2 is added to achieve a final concentration of 0.1 % trypsin. As with the CSF for culture, an increased volume aids detection. The treated sample is then vortexed and then incubated at 37°C for 30 minutes. Following incubation, the sample is again vortexed and centrifuged for 45–60 minutes at 12,000 × gravity in a microcentrifuge.

The pellet is resuspended in 20 μl of lysis buffer 0.5 percent sodium dodecylsulfate (SDS), 1 percent NP40, 0.2 M NaCl, 10 μM dithiothreitol (DTT), 10 mM EDTA, 20 mM Tris-HCl at pH 7.5. The DTT is essential for efficient DNA extraction because reducing agents are known to disrupt disulfide bond in the outer membrane of *Chlamydia* sp. [9] and thus allow better access of a non-specific protease to peptide bonds. To this lysis mixture is added 8 μl of Proteinase K 20 mg/l (Boehringer-Mannheim, Indianapolis, IN). The specimen is mixed and incubated overnight at 37°C. Initial extraction of this specimen is performed with a mixture of phenol:chloroform:isoamyl alcohol 25:24:1 (Sigma) followed by 2 extractions with chloroform. Purified DNA is then extracted from the aqueous fraction of this specimen with Na acetate 1:10 dilution by volume of a 3 M solution (Fisher Scientific, Pittsburgh, PA). This is done using a mixing/precipitation procedure with 2:2.5 dilution by volume of cold absolute ethanol. The DNA is washed with 70 percent ethanol in water, spun 600 × gravity for 5 minutes at ambient temperature, and resuspended in 20 μl of water.

PCR is performed by amplifying the entire MOMP gene (~1.2 kb) using Deep Vent or Vent polymerase (New England Biolabs [NEB], Boston, MA) in the manufacturer's buffer with no additional $MgCl_2$. Other polymerases are either inactive or less efficient for amplification of this gene. The specific MOMP primers used are: MOMP forward-ATG AAA AAA CTC TTA AAG TCG GCG TTA TTA TCC GCC GC, and MOMP reverse-TTA GAA TCT GAA CTG ACC AGA TAC GTG AGC AGC TCT CTC G. The reaction mixtures contain 20 μl of target DNA, 200 picoMoles of each primer, 200 μM each dNTP, and 1 unit of Deep Vent or Vent polymerase NEB. The PCR reaction is carried out for 35 cycles at 94°C for 1 minute, 58°C for 2 minutes, and 74°C for 3 minutes. PCR reactions are analyzed by electrophoresis in 1 % agarose gel for 45 minutes at 95 volts with ethidium bromide detection of a 1.2 kb band. For conformation and increased sensitivity of the PCR assay, a Southern hybridization is done. This method uses a digoxigenin-labeled DIG (Boehringer-Mannheim) full-length MOMP probe from the TWAR stain of *C. pneumoniae* VR-1310 (American Type Culture Collection [ATCC], Manassas, VA) and confirms the PCR signal as well as allows visualization of some PCR signals not visible by ethidium bromide of agarose gels.

Southern hybridization of full-length MOMP gene product

Southern hybridization was done using modifications of a published method [3] as follows: First, a digoxigenin-labeled probe for the full-length MOMP gene product is made using the TWAR strain of *C. pneumoniae* VR-1310 (ATCC). After the full-length MOMP gene of the TWAR strain is amplified by PCR as described above, the full-length MOMP product is electrophoresed in low melting point agarose gel at 95 V for 60 minutes. The full-length PCR band is cut from the gel and placed in a separate microcentrifuge tube with the addition of sterile distilled water to a ratio of 3 ml of water to 1 gram of gel. The tube is boiled for 10 minutes at 100°C, cooled to 37°C, and labeled with DIG as detailed by the kit's manufacturer (Boehringer-Mannheim). This probe is used to confirm the full-length PCR product as follows: The agarose gels from the full-length PCR products are treated with 0.4M NaOH for 20 minutes and the DNA transferred by capillary blotting to positively charged nylon membranes. Membranes are pre-hybridized in hybridization buffer 10 % Dextran sulfate, 1 M NaCl, 1 % SDS for at least 60 minutes at 65°C. The full-length PCR DIG-labeled probe 100 ng is added in fresh hybridization buffer and incubated at 65°C overnight. Blots are washed 3 times in 2X SSC,

1 % SDS at ambient temperature, and an additional three times with 1X SSC, 0.1 % SDS at 65°C. Finally, three high stringency washes are performed in 0.1X SSC, 0.1 % SDS at ambient temperature. Membranes are blocked in 5 % w/v dehydrated non-fat milk in PBS with 0.2 % Tween 20 for 60 minutes at ambient temperature. The membranes are then incubated in anti-DIG-alkaline phosphatase conjugated Fab fragments diluted 1:5000 in PBS containing 0.2 % Tween 20, washed three times in PBS/0.2 % Tween 20, and developed with NBT/BCIP substrate (Boehringer-Mannheim).

Nested PCR confirmation of MOMP gene

Although nested PCR was not reported in the initial study [26], we have developed and now include a nested PCR procedure. Nested PCR primers were chosen in variable domains 1 and 4 within the MOMP gene that provided additional specificity for *C. pneumoniae* and yielded a 727 base pair band. These primers are: Nest MOMP forward-GCT GCT GCA AAC TAT ACT ACT GCC, Nest MOMP reverse-GAA TCA GTA GTA GAC AAT GCT GTG G. The target for the nested primers is 5 µl of PCR product from the full length MOMP PCR reaction. The nested PCR reaction is carried out under the same buffer and reagent conditions used for the full length MOMP. These are 35 cycles at 94°C for 1 minute, 45°C for 2 minutes, and 72°C for 3 minutes, including a 7 minute final extension at 72°C. PCR reactions were analyzed by electrophoresis in 1 % agarose gel for 45 minutes at 95 volts. For confirmation and enhanced sensitivity of the nested PCR, the nested PCR gels may be analyzed also by Southern hybridization.

Southern hybridization of nested MOMP gene product

Southern hybridization of the nested MOMP gene product is done in the same way used for full-length MOMP with one difference as follows. After the full-length MOMP gene of the TWAR strain is amplified, 5 µl of this product is used as target for a nested PCR reaction. The nested MOMP product is electrophoresed in low melting point agarose gel at 95 V for 60 minutes. The nested PCR band is cut from the gel and placed in a separate microcentrifuge tube with the addition of sterile distilled water in a ratio of 3 ml of water to 1 gram of gel. The tube is boiled for 10 minutes at 100°C, cooled to 37°C, and labeled with DIG as detailed by the kit's manufacturer (Boehringer-Mannheim). This probe is used to confirm the nested PCR product as follows: The agarose gel with nested PCR product is treated with 0.4 M NaOH for 20 minutes and the DNA transferred by capillary blotting to positively charged nylon membranes. The rest of the procedure is identical to that for the full-length MOMP except the nested PCR DIG-labeled probe 100 ng is used.

ELISA measurement of antibody levels in CSF to EB antigens of C. pneumoniae

CSF antibodies to *C. pneumoniae* are measured by an ELISA technique modified from a published procedure [19] as follows: 96-well plates are coated with 100 μl of *C. pneumoniae* EB antigens 250 ng/well. EB antigens are prepared from concentrated *C. pneumoniae* EBs by first treating them with 25 mM DTT, 2 % 2-mercaptoethanol, and 2 % SDS for 5 minutes at 100°C. These treated EBs are then sonicated, centrifuged 500 × g for 30 minutes at room temperature and resuspended 2 mg/l protein in PBS pH 7.4.

Concentrated *C. pneumoniae* EBs are obtained by growing *C. pneumoniae* ATTC VR-1310 in 25 ml flasks containing a confluent growth of HL cells (WRF) in Dulbecco's minimal essential medium DMEM (GIBCO) and 10 % FCS. Infection is facilitated by two washes with HBSS followed by a 20 minute preincubation with DEAE-Dextran 30 μg/ml in HBSS. The infectious inoculum is added to the flasks in a 2 ml volume of serum-free media. The flasks are then centrifuged at 1,200 × gravity for 1 hour at 4°C. To the spun flasks is added 2 ml of Iscoves medium containing 4 mg/l cyclohexamide, 20 % FCS, 4 mM L-glutamine, and 100 mg/l gentamicin. The flasks are then incubated at 37°C for 3 days at which time the infected cells begin to lyse and release EBs. On day 4, the culture flasks are sonicated for 20 seconds, and the cell debris removed by centrifugation at 600 × gravity for 5 minutes at room temperature. The supernatant containing the infectious EBs is centrifuged at 18,000 × gravity for 30 minutes and the pellet resolubilized in water containing 25 mM DTT, 2 % 2-mercaptoethanol, and 2 % SDS.

After the EB antigens are added to the 96-well plate, the plates are incubated overnight and then unoccupied sites in the wells blocked with 1 % BSA, PBS-Tween 20 for 60 minutes. The CSF samples are added to each well in a final concentration of 1 μg of immunoglobulin diluted in 100 μl of PBS as determined by rate laser nephelometric methods, Behring Nephelometer Analyzer II (Behring Diagnostics Inc, San Jose, CA). The plates are incubated overnight at 4°C after which they were washed with PBS-Tween 20. Next, peroxidase-conjugated goat anti-human IgG 1:10,000 (Sigma) is added. Following incubation for 2 hours, the plates are washed with PBS-Tween 20 and the substrate added. The absorbance units at 405 nm are read using an ELISA reader (Bio-Tech Instruments, Burlington, VT) at 60 minutes.

Western blot assays of EB antigens reactive against CSF immunoglobulins

Western blot assays against CSF immunoglobulins are performed using modifications from a published method [5] as follows: EB antigens are prepared from concentrated *C. pneumoniae* EBs by treating them with 25 mM DTT, 2 % 2-mercaptoethanol, and 2 % SDS for 5 min at 100°C as done for the ELISA procedure. Treated EBs are sonicated, and then 2.5 μg of the sonicated protein is loaded in each well and run on an 8 % SDS PAGE gel at 100V for 2 hours at ambient temperature. The gel is transferred to nitrocellulose membrane at 100V for 1 hour at ambient temperature. Individual strips are cut and incubated in 3 % BSA-tris-buffered saline with Tween 20 (TBST) for 2 hours at ambient temperature to block unoccupied sites. The strips are then washed three times with TBST. CSF containing 5 µg of immunoglobulin is added to the strips, and they are incubated for two days at 4°C. Following this incubation with CSF, the strips are washed three times with TBST and again incubated with peroxidase-conjugated goat anti-human IgG 1:500 (Sigma) for 90 minutes at ambient temperature. Finally, the strips are examined using a chemiluminiscent detection assay (Pierce, Rockford, IL). Control experiments use cell lysates of uninfected HL cells instead of *C. pneumoniae* EBs in Western blot assays.

Isoelectric focusing/Western blot assays for CSF immunoglobulins

Isoelectric focusing/Western blot assays for CSF immunoglobulins were performed using modifications from a published method [4, 5] as follows: Isoelectric focusing (IEF) is performed with 0.2 µg of immunoglobulin from CSF obtained from MS patients and OND controls. Focusing is carried out under constant voltage conditions in a stepped fashion (100V for 15 min, 200V for 15 min, and 450V for 20 min). The IEF gel is transferred to nitrocellulose paper (Bio-Rad, Transblot, 0.45 µm) that was precoated with *C. pneumoniae* EB antigens by overnight incubation with gentle rocking at 4°C. EB antigens are prepared as described from concentrated *C. pneumoniae* EBs that are treated with 25 mM DTT, 2 % 2-mercaptoethanol, and 2 % SDS for 5 minutes at 100°C and then sonicated, centrifuged 500 × gravity for 30 minutes at room temperature and resuspended 2 mg/l protein in PBS pH 7.4. Unoccupied sites are blocked with 3 % BSA. Antibody bound to antigen is probed with peroxidase-conjugated goat anti-human IgG (Sigma) using a chemiluminescent detection assay (Pierce).

Results

Our initial study [26] evaluated 17 patients with reactive remitting MS 4M/13F (mean age 31 years at the time of diagnosis of clinically definite disease) and 20 patients with progressive MS 10M/10F (mean age 40 years). All except 5 of these 37 MS patients had oligoclonal bands in the CSF.

Twenty-seven patients 12M/15F (mean age 39 years) with other neurological diseases (OND) were selected as controls. Of these, 19 had CSF abnormalities i.e., increased CSF protein and/or increase in CSF lymphocytes consistent with either a break in the blood–CSF or blood–brain barrier. One patient with chronic meningitis of unknown etiology had oligoclonal bands in the CSF. Of the remaining 7 OND control patients with normal CSF profiles, two were diagnosed with cerebrovascular disease and one case each was seen with brain abscess, Hashimoto's encephalopathy, polyneuropathy, Wernicke-Korsakow's encephalopathy and a syndrome consistent with vasculitis and stroke.

Direct evidence for the presence of *C. pneumoniae* in the CNS was determined by CSF cultures. Among patients with newly diagnosed relapsing remitting MS,

47 % of patients (8/17) had *C. pneumoniae* isolated from CSF cultures. Figure 1 shows representative positive and negative culture results. Among patients with progressive MS, 80 % of patients 16/20) were culture positive. Figure 2 shows a DFA stain from CSF for *C. pneumoniae*.

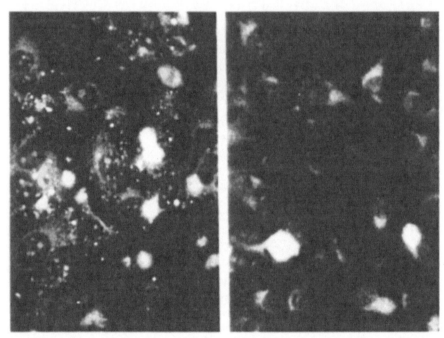

Figure 1. HL cells stained for chlamydial inclusions with *C. pneumoniae*-specific fluoresceine-conjugated mouse monoclonal antibody and Evan's blue counterstain. Left: HL cells inoculated with CSF from an MS patient clearly showing fluorescent inclusions following 7 days of incubation. Right: HL cells inoculated with CSF from an OND patient showing no fluorescent inclusions. These cultures were reported as culture-positive and culture-negative for *C. pneumoniae*.

In contrast, *C. pneumoniae* was isolated from CSF in only 3 OND control patients. One of these three patients was diagnosed as having post infectious encephalomyelitis (PIE), which may, in fact, represent a variant of MS. The remaining two patients presented with inflammatory myelopathy; one of these being of unknown etiology and the other thought to be due to HSV-2. In these latter two patients, changes consistent with inflammatory myelopathy were seen on MRIs of the spinal cords.

The presence of *C. pneumoniae* in the CNS was also evaluated by PCR methods. This method assayed CSF for the major outer membrane protein (MOMP) gene of *C. pneumoniae*. The specific 1.2 kb band for the MOMP gene seen following ethidium bromide staining of agarose gels was confirmed using a Southern hybridization method in which DIG-labeled MOMP gene probes were used. Figure 3 demonstrates a representative PCR/Southern hybridization result. The MOMP gene for *C. pneumoniae* was amplified and confirmed in all 17 (100 %)

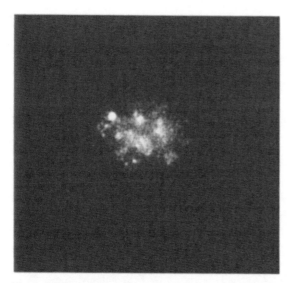

Figure 2. Direct fluorescent antibody stain of *C. pneumoniae* from Cytospin-concentrated CSF of an MS patient.

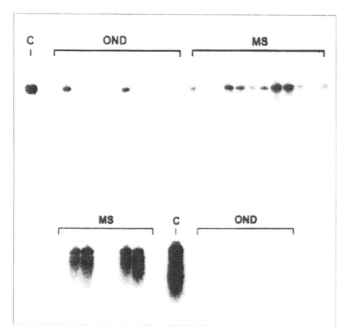

Figure 3. Representative PCR amplification for the presence of MOMP gene in the CSF of MS patients versus OND controls. Lane C represents PCR products from EBs of the ATCC VR-1310 strain of *C. pneumoniae* that served as a positive internal control. The bands represent the 1.2 Kb MOMP gene. DNA was amplified with MOMP primers and then probed with digoxigenin-labeled MOMP probe. Three positive signals were noted in the OND group; two in the upper panel and one in the lower panel.

relapsing remitting MS patients and 19 of 20 (95 %) of progressive MS patients versus 5 of 27 (18 %) OND controls. One progressive MS patient and one control were negative for the MOMP gene, but were positive by culture. Of the five OND control patients who were positive for the MOMP gene, three had thoracic myelitis; the fourth had acute inflammatory demyelinating polyneuropathy (AIDP), while the fifth had a stroke. In both groups of relapsing remitting and progressive MS patients, all culture-negative MS patients were positive by PCR/Southern hybridization assays.

Indirect evidence of *C. pneumoniae* infection in the CNS was determined by the detection of CSF antibodies against preparations of *C. pneumoniae* elementary bodies that were reduced/solublized/sonicated in order to produce EB antigens. An ELISA method was used to detect CSF antibodies against these EB antigens. To ensure that differences in the ELISA absorbance signal was not due to differences in the concentration of antibodies in the CSF, the amount of immunoglobulins in CSF was determined by rate laser nephelometric methods in order to add equal amounts to the ELISA plates. Mean absorbance OD values for antibody response to EB antigens using CSF from 17 relapsing remitting MS patients was 0.185 ± 0.042 while the mean OD in the control OND group was 0.078 ± 0.025 ($p<0.01$ Fisher's test). Of 17 patients with relapsing remitting MS, 15 patients (88 %) had OD values that were three standard deviations from values in the OND group. The mean OD of 20 progressive MS patients was 0.237 ± 0.11, while in the OND control group it was 0.093 ± 0.022 ($p<0.001$ Fisher's test). Seventeen of 20 (85 %) MS patients tested had absorbance values in CSF that were three standard deviations greater than those seen in the control group. Overall, 86 % of MS patients studied had absorbance values in CSF that were three standard deviations greater than those seen in the OND control group. These observations suggest that increased CSF antibodies against *C. pneumoniae* may be present in the majority of patients with MS.

The specificity of the CSF antibodies was evaluated by a modified Western blot assay that used EB antigens. Figure 4 demonstrates a representative Western blot assay. Equal amounts of CSF immunoglobulins were incubated with EB antigens in order to control for differences in immunoglobulin concentrations in the CSF. Seventeen of 20 CSF samples from MS patients demonstrated prominent reactivity to a 75kD protein of *C. pneumoniae* with weaker reactivity to 65kD, 60kD, and 55kD proteins observed in 13 of these 20 MS patients. In 19 of these 20 MS patients, the strength of the bands seen on Western blot correlated with the ELISA OD units. In contrast, reactivity to this 75kD protein was seen in only 4 of 20 OND controls. In all 4, the reactivity was weak when compared to MS patients. One of these OND control with PIE was culture-positive for *C. pneumoniae*. Another patient with AIDP was positive by PCR/Southern hybridization to *C. pneumoniae* but culture-negative. The other two OND controls with positive Western blots were negative for *C. pneumoniae* by culture and PCR/Southern hybridization.

When Western blots were performed using cytosolic lysates from uninfected HL cells, no binding of antibody was seen in either the MS patient or the OND

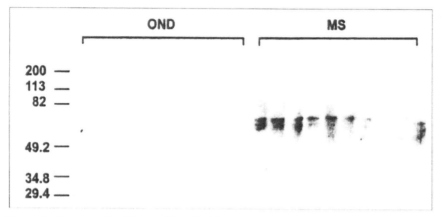

Figure 4. Representative Western blot visualization of CSF immunoglobulins reactive to EB antigens of *C. pneumoniae* in MS patients and OND controls.

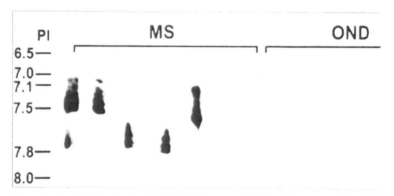

Figure 5. Specificity of oligoclonal CFS immunoglobulins demonstrated by IEF/Western blot studies to EB antigens of *C. pneumoniae*. The blots are from a representative group of 5 MS patients and 5 OND controls.

group, suggesting that the antibody binding was specific for elementary body antigens of *C. pneumoniae*.

MS patients are known to have an increase in CSF immunoglobulins in which a portion of this increase is seen as oligoclonal bands on isoelectric focusing gels. These oligoclonal bands represent cationic antibodies that have isoelectric points in the anodic region of the gel. The presence of these cationic antibodies in the CSF was evaluated using a procedure in which isoelectric focusing (IEF) of CSF is followed by Western blot assays using EB antigens. Of 20 progressive MS patients studied to date, 12 have CSF immunoglobulins at isoelectric points of 7.5 or greater that react with EB antigens Figure 5 shows a representative IEF / Western blot result. The lack of anti-chlamydial immunoglobulins in IEF / Western gels in some patients who have oligoclonal bands and positive PCR/Southern hybridization assays may relate to differences in the affinity of antibodies to linear antigen displayed on the membrane. Two OND control patients, one positive by culture and the other by PCR/Southern hybridization, demonstrated similar cationic antibodies against EB antigens. These results suggest that cationic antichlamydial antibodies are present in the CSF of patients with MS and represent, in part, the specificity for the characteristic oligoclonal bands seen in MS.

Discussion

Association of *Chlamydia* species with neurological disorders has been noted [1, 8, 10, 14, 15]. Further evaluation of the possible association of *C. pneumoniae* with MS was prompted by our initial observation of *C. pneumoniae* infection of the CNS associated with MS [27]. In this initial case, routine culture methods for isolation of *Chlamydia* were used [21, 24]. Briefly, this method started with a large volume of CSF 5 ml that was first centrifuged (Centra-8R; IEC) at ambient temperature for 1 hour at 4,500 × gravity in order to concentrate any EBs. This spun sediment was then inoculated in duplicate onto HL cell (WRF) monolayers in shell vials. These shell vials were centrifuged in a swinging bucket rotor at ambient temperature for 1 hour at 1,800 × gravity in order to deposit the inoculated specimen onto the cell monolayer. Following this inoculation, media containing cyclohexamide was added to these shell vials, and they were incubated with for 3 days at 37°C. Finally, the cell monolayers were stained with a fluoresceine-tagged monoclonal antibody (WRF) against *C. pneumoniae* and examined for inclusions by immunofluorescent microscopy (Nikon).

Although this routine chlamydial culture method was sufficient in our first patient, we felt that a more thorough evaluation should use a protocol that allows concentration of potential EBs from small volumes of CSF. In addition, this protocol should provide optimal cell culture conditions in order to maximize isolation of this organism. The protocol should also be able to detect and amplify *C. pneumoniae* DNA in the CSF. Finally, this protocol should assess the CNS humoral response to *C. pneumoniae*. Accordingly, we developed a protocol designed to enhance the recovery of *C. pneumoniae* from CSF, to assay for DNA by PCR, and to measure the CSF humoral immune response to this pathogen [26]. Using this optimized protocol, our initial study [26] suggests that infection of CNS with *C. pneumoniae* is present in patients with newly diagnosed relapsing remitting MS as well as in patients with progressive MS, but not in OND controls. The most striking evidence for CNS infection with *C. pneumoniae* is the isolation of this pathogen from CSF in 64% of all MS patients (24/37). The reason for the increased detection of *C. pneumoniae* by culture in progressive MS patients over that with relapsing remitting MS is not certain, but may relate to an increased burden of disease or an increased involvement of the spinal cord and therefore easier detection in the spinal fluid.

At least 19 of 27 patients in the OND control group had inflammatory diseases that were restricted to the CNS as evidenced by the abnormalities in the CSF and served as appropriate controls for the study. In this control group, one patient with AIDP had a positive PCR/Southern hybridization assay for the MOMP gene as well as CSF antibodies against *C. pneumoniae*. *C. pneumoniae* has been reported as one of the causes of AIDP [10]. Another OND control patient with a stroke had a positive PCR/S assay for the MOMP gene; *C. pneumoniae* has been isolated from CNS vessels and has been associated with cerebrovascular disease [8, 31]. One patient with PIE had inflammatory disease of the white matter, but was included in the OND control group since she did not satisfy the clinical criteria for MS.

In the three patients with inflammatory myelopathies two were PCR and culture positive while one was only weakly PCR positive. It is not clear whether the neurologic syndromes in these patients represent the initial attack of MS. If that were the case, it would further substantiate our hypothesis that infection of CNS with *C. pneumoniae* occurs early and persists throughout the course of the disease.

In summary, evidence for *C. pneumoniae* infection of the CNS was found in all patients with MS that were studied [26]. These results do not establish a causal relationship between *C. pneumoniae* infection of the CNS and the development of MS. In fact, there is no current evidence for *C. pneumoniae* causing CNS demyelinating disease and axon loss. However, it is interesting to note that two agents currently in use for the therapy of MS, beta-interferon and methotrexate, inhibit the replication of Chlamydia *in vitro* [11, 30].

C. pneumoniae is a common respiratory pathogen and serologic evidence of infection is present in significant portion of the population [12, 18, 19]. Seroconversion generally begins in the first decade of life with a majority of individuals showing immunological evidence of exposure by the fourth decade [12, 18]. Since a large number of individuals are infected with the organism, it is possible that *C. pneumoniae* is the inciting agent of MS in genetically susceptible individuals. The organism may provide an initial inflammatory insult as well as a chronic stimulus, thereby establishing a chronic state of immune activation. Conversely, CNS infection by *C. pneumoniae* in MS patients may simply represent a secondary infection of damaged CNS tissue. *C. pneumoniae* is well known to infect macrophages and monocytes as well as endothelial and smooth muscle cells of blood vessels [8]. This pathogen thus could be transported to inflamed CNS tissues by infected monocytes/macrophages [23, 32] that were responding to an initial triggering event. This triggering event could be an acute viral infection or autoimmune reaction. Regardless of the exact role of *C. pneumoniae* in patients with MS, our study demonstrates a strong association between these two entities. A well-designed therapeutic trial directed at eliminating *C. pneumoniae* from the CNS may provide additional answers regarding the role of the organism in the pathogenesis of MS [25].

References

1. Balin BJ, Gerad HC, Arking EJ, et al. (1998) Identification and localization of *Chlamydia pneumoniae* in the Alzheimer's brain. Med Microbiol Immunol 187: 23–42
2. Cles LD, Bruch K, Stamm WE (1990) Use of HL cells for improved isolation and passage of *Chlamydia pneumoniae*. J Clin Microbiol 28: 938–940
3. Dalhoff K, Maass M (1996) *Chlamydia pneumoniae* in hospitalized patients. Clinical characteristic and diagnostic value of polymerase chain reaction detection in BAL. Chest 110: 351–356

4. Dorries R, Muelen VL (1984) Detection and identification of virus specific oligoclonal IgG in unconcentrated CSF by immunoblot. J Neuroimmunol 7: 77–89
5. Friedank HM, Herr AS, Jacobs E (1993) Identification of *Chlamydia pneumoniae*-specific protein antigens in immunoblots. Eur J Microbiol Infect Dis 12: 947–951
6. Gaydos CA, Eiden JJ, Oldbach D, et al. (1994) Diagnosis of *Chlamydia pneumoniae* infection in patients with community-acquired pneumonia by polymerase chain reaction enzyme immunoassay. Clin Infect Dis 19: 157–160
7. Gaydos CA, Summersgill JT, Sahney N, Ramirez JA, Quinn TC (1996) Replication of *Chlamydia pneumoniae* in vitro in human macrophages, endothelial cells, and aortic artery smooth muscle cells. Infect Immun 64: 1614–1620
8. Grayston JT, Ku CC, Coulson AS, et al. (1995) *Chlamydia pneumoniae* (TWAR) in atherosclerosis of the carotid artery. Circulation 92: 3397–3400
9. Hackstadt T, Todd WJ, Caldwell HD (1985) Disulfide-mediated interactions of the chlamydial major outer membrane protein: role in the differentiation of chlamydiae. J Bacteriol 161: 25–31
10. Haidl S, Ivarsson S, Bjerre I, Persson K (1992) Guillain-Barré syndrome after *Chlamydia pneumoniae* infection. N Engl J Med 326: 576–577
11. Hanna L, Merigan TC, Jawetz F (1966) Inhibition of TRIC agents by virus induced interferon. Proc Soc Exp Med Biol 122: 417–421
12. Kauppinen M, Saikku P (1995) Pneumonia due to *Chlamydia pneumoniae:* prevalence, clinical features, diagnosis, and treatment. Clin Infect Dis 21 (Suppl 3): S244–S252
13. Kazuyama Y, Lee SM, Amamiya K, Taguchi F (1997) A novel method for isolation of *Chlamydia pneumoniae* by treatment with trypsin or EDTA. J Clin Microbiol 35: 1624–1626
14. Korman TM, Turnidge JD, Grayson ML (1997) Neurologic complications of chlamydial infections: case report and review. Clin Infect Dis 25: 847–851
15. Koskiniemi M, Gencay M, Salonen O, Puolakkainen M, Farkkila M, Saikku P, Vaheri P (1996) *Chlamydia pneumoniae* associated with CNS infections. Eur J Neurol 36: 160–163
16. Kuo CC, Grayston JT (1990) A sensitive cell line, HL cells, for isolation and propagation of *Chlamydia pneumoniae* strain TWAR. J Infect Dis 162: 755–758
17. Kuo CC, Grayston JT (1988) Factors affecting variability and growth in HeLa 229 cells of *Chlamydia* sp. strain TWAR. J Clin Microbiol 26: 812–815
18. Kuo CC, Jackson LA, Campbell LA, Grayston JT (1995) *Chlamydia pneumoniae* (TWAR). Clin Microbiol Rev 8: 451–461
19. Ladany S, Black CM, Farshy CE, Ossewaarde JM, Barnes RC (1989) Enzyme immunoassay to determine exposure to *Chlamydia pneumoniae* strain (TWAR). J Clin Microbiol 27: 2778–2783
20. Maass M, Harig U (1994) Comparison of sample preparation methods for detection of *Chlamydia pneumoniae* in bronchoalveolar lavage fluid by PCR. J Clin Microbiol 32 (10): 2616–2619
21. Maass M, Harig U (1995) Evaluation of culture conditions used for isolation of *Chlamydia pneumoniae*. Am J Clin Pathol 103: 141–148
22. Melgosa-Perez PM, Kuo CC, Campbell LA (1991) Sequence analysis of the major outer membrane protein gene of *Chlamydia pneumoniae*. Infect Immun 59: 2195–2199
23. Moazed TC, Kuo CC, Grayston JT, Campbell LA (1998) Evidence of systemic dissemination of *Chlamydia pneumoniae* via macrophages in the mouse. J Infect Dis 177: 1322–1325

24. Schachter J, Stamm W (1995) *Chlamydia*. In: Murray PR, Baron EJ, Pfaller MA, Tenover FC, Yolken RH (eds) Manual of Clinical Microbiology. ASM Press, Washington, p 672
25. Sriram S (1997) Future of MS therapeutics: rational approach targeting putative pathogenic mechanisms. In: Goodkind D, Rudick R (eds) MS: Advances in Trial Design and Therapeutics. Springer, New York, pp 47–62
26. Sriram S, Stratton CW, Yao S, Tharp A, Ding L, Bannan JD, Mitchell WM (1999) *Chlamydia pneumoniae* infection of the CNS in multiple sclerosis. Ann Neurol 46: 6–14
27. Sriram S, Mitchell W, Stratton C (1998) Multiple sclerosis associated with *Chlamydia pneumoniae* infection of the CNS. Neurology 50: 571–572
28. Theunissen JJH, van Heijst BYM, Wagenvoort JHT, Stolz E, Michel MF (1992) Factors influencing the infectivity of *Chlamydia pneumoniae* elementary bodies on HL cells. J Clin Microbiol 30: 1388–1391
29. Tjhie JHT, Roosendaal R, MacLaren DM, Vandenbroucke-Gauls CMJE (1997) Improvement of growth of *Chlamydia pneumoniae* on Hep-2 cells by pretreatment with polyethylene glycol in combination with additional centrifugation and extension of culture time. J Clin Microbiol 35: 1883–1884
30. Wang LL, Henson E, McClarty G (1994) Characterization of trimethoprim- and sulphisoxazole-resistant *Chlamydia trachomatis*. Molecular Microbiol 14: 271–281
31. Wimmer MLJ, Sandmann-Strupp R, Saikku P, Haberl RL (1996) Association of chlamydial infection with cerebrovascular disease. Stroke 27: 2207–2210
32. Yang ZP, Kuo CC, Grayston JT (1995) Systemic dissemination of *Chlamydia pneumoniae* following intranasal inoculation in mice. J Infect Dis 171: 736–738

Discussion

Anonymus:
In multiple sclerosis you very often find also antibodies against viruses like rubella, measles and mumps, also HHV6. How do you combine this view that you find antibodies against viruses and maybe antibodies against Chlamydia as well?

Stratton:
If we just had the antibody data, I wouldn't be standing here. We got culture data and PCR data which, to me, is compelling.

Boman:
I have read your case report in *Neurology* in February and found this very interesting. So I decided to have a look at multiple sclerosis. We have an MS clinic at our hospital and I got 150 CSF, 1 ml from each patient and control, so patient-to-control ratio was 1:1. For 50 of them we used exactly the same procedure as you have with DTT, centrifugation etc. and all were negative. Then we looked at 100 with our routine method for viral agents like herpes simplex with a commercial kit from Qiagen, all were negative. Then we sent 100 of these to Dr. Hammerschlag for culture attempts and all were negative. Then the question was, do these patients have a intrathecal antibody production? From 64 of them we have simultaneously collected serum and CSF and all but one were normal, one was a borderline with a ratio 1:64 which is not pathologic but also not normal.

All the others, the MS patients and the controls, were normal. I think these are quite divergent results.

Stratton:
I am aware of Jens' work and there are obviously problems with detecting or not detecting Chlamydia. All I can say at this point is, the absence of proof is not proof of absence. When others have looked and perhaps found them or not found it, we will have a better understanding.

Byrne:
It might be helpful, too, if you could actually show cultural data, photographs of your inclusions. I think if you want to really get a critical appraisal of the community, then you need to show the data so that we can look at it.

Stratton:
That will be in the paper coming out soon.

Boman:
I went to the lab in Vanderbilt just to see the cultures and unfortunately you didn't have any positive cultures. You had some photographs but it didn't look like chlamydial inclusions. I must admit that I am a little skeptical to the cultures.

Stratton:
They look like Chlamydia inclusions in one published article in the Chlamydia book from Italy. They also look like Chlamydia inclusions that we have with control ATCC elementary bodies. We have also sequenced a number of these and have done everything to determine whether it is Chlamydia or not.

Stille:
In my opinion there are epidemiological arguments which hint that Chlamydia and MS might be in connection. One argument is the so-called Faroer studies. An epidemic on the Faroers was analyzed and a potential pathogen was defined. The characteristic of the potential pathogen fits perfectly *C. pneumoniae* which was at that time not yet known, for they defined the pathogen around 1984 just before the finding of *C. pneumoniae*. It has to be kept in mind that atherosclerosis and multiple sclerosis have the same funny type of geographic epidemiology. There are countries with high incidence of atherosclerosis and also high incidence of multiple sclerosis, so maybe there are epidemiological hints. It has to be kept in mind that intravascular infections usually lead to infections of the brain, at least in some percentage.

Leinonen:
But still I think that there is much more evidence on the association of *C. pneumoniae* with atherosclerosis than with multiple sclerosis.

Chapter 4
Epidemiology and Public Health Impacts of *Chlamydia pneumoniae* Infections

4.1
Trends and variations of chronic diseases in populations – Can infectious agents help to solve the puzzles?

H.W. Hense

The reason for our scientific focus on cardiovascular disease and atherosclerosis lies in its nature as a phenomenon of entire populations, in its mass dimension. These diseases do not occur in just a few individuals but every year, repeatedly and predictably, in hundreds of thousands of subjects in our populations. Chronic disease epidemiologists are trying to understand the determinants of these processes and attempt to dissect their trends and variations in differing populations. A new hypothesis, such as that of infectious agents causing or triggering cardiovascular events, is always greeted with great expectations as there are still major puzzles to solve in cardiovascular disease (CVD) epidemiology. In this presentation, I will try to sketch just a few of the puzzles that we encounter on the population level and I will continue into a rather personal view of the potentials which the infection hypothesis may offer to help solve these puzzles.

First, I would like to characterize the magnitude of the epidemic. Such an epidemic of chronic diseases can best be assessed by looking at the total numbers of deaths and diseased from CVD, at the variation of these numbers, and at temporal trends. The first table (Table 1) is an overview of the age-standardized mortality in 1994 for men and women aged 30 to 69 years in some European countries. Results are based on official vital statistics and it is obvious that in terms of all-cause mortality some countries are definitely worse off than others. The countries are ranked according to their mortality rates of all cardiovascular diseases which includes ischemic heart disease, coronary heart disease, cerebrovascular disease and other types of heart diseases. It becomes clear that in populations with a high all-cause mortality the mortality of cardiovascular diseases is high as well. This can be expressed as a proportionate CVD mortality which reflects the percentage of deaths per year attributable to CVD. Apparently, countries with high total mortality have a disproportionately high CVD death rate and the proportionate CVD mortality ranges from over 40 % in Hungary or Finland down to 20 % in the Mediterranean countries. This pattern is also observed in women although on a lower absolute level. We summarize that, in general, people living in populations with high death rates die more frequently from CVD. We may ask for the first time, can this be explained by infectious agents?

Table 1. Age-standardized mortality rates per 100,000 in Europe 1990: all causes and cardiovascular diseases (CVD), proportionate mortality of CVD (in %).

	Men, 30 to 69 years.		Women, 30 to 69 years.	
ICD-9:	All causes 001 – 999	Cardiovascular 390 – 458	All causes 001 – 999	Cardiovascular 390 – 458
Hungary	1,616	648 (40 %)	688	273 (40 %)
Poland	1,395	598 (43 %)	558	230 (41 %)
Finland	958	424 (44 %)	371	122 (33 %)
Germany (East)	1,098	418 (38 %)	520	180 (35 %)
Germany (West)	796	283 (36 %)	383	103 (27 %)
Italy	705	207 (29 %)	320	80 (25 %)
Spain	717	193 (27 %)	297	74 (25 %)
France	782	163 (21 %)	306	53 (17 %)

Source: WHO 1994

On the other hand, it is often claimed that mortality data are not reliable, that there is misclassification due to varying coding rules or insufficient clinical knowledge of the person filling out the death certificates. We addressed this problem, among many others, in a large international collaborative study, the WHO MONICA-Project [1]. There were many centers worldwide working with a common protocol to register all cases of coronary heart disease occurring in the population. Therefore, the MONICA project can present representative CHD morbidity data that can be validly compared between countries [2]. The first figure (Figure 1) confirms that there are also large variations in CVD morbidity rates between populations and that what has been shown for mortality holds also true for morbidity rates. Moreover, the populations of Finland or the eastern European countries show high rates whereas down at the bottom there are the populations of southern Europe and, in particular, those from Asia (the Beijing center is an example). Of note, the within-country differences are much less pronounced than those between national samples.

But we do not only have differences in the magnitude of population rates but we also have differences in their changes with time. Figure 2 shows time trends of CVD mortality between 1979 and 1993. In many populations with high CVD rates, like for example, Hungary and Poland, we observed fairly constant or even slightly rising trends. By contrast, Finland which started with very high rates back in the 1970's – actually the highest in Europe at that time – demonstrated dramatic mortality declines of 36% over this time period. Interestingly, Italy, Spain and France, starting already at a low level, still had some decline in their mortality rates. The reasons for these divergent trends are not very clear. One pattern seems to be that the central and Eastern European countries show rising CVD mortality rates whereas the industrialized Western countries generally exhibit declining rates of similar magnitude. As for the Asian countries mentioned above, some are characterized by very low coronary heart disease rates and at the same time high cerebrovascular disease rates. Nevertheless, despite their low CHD rates, countries like Japan showed still declining rates over the last two decades. For the high cerebrovascular disease rates the downward trends were even stronger.

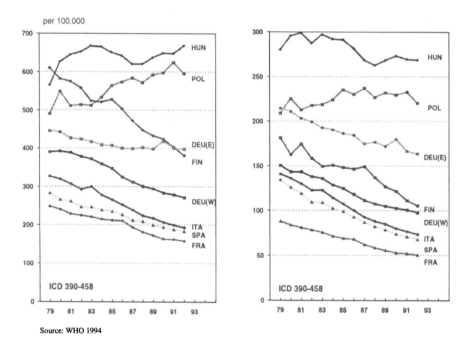

Figure 1. Age-adjusted annual coronary event rates (per 100,000) in men and women, 35 to 64 years. From reference [2].

In summary, epidemiological evidence indicates that morbidity and mortality of CVD rise with age, that rates in men are consistently higher than in women, that these diseases are very common in industrialized countries but with large differences between countries. We find major time trends and these trends are divergent over the last decades. Can we find any explanations or reasons for this puzzling picture?

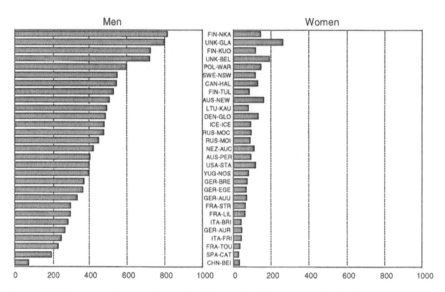

Figure 2. Time trends for age-adjusted cardiovascular disease mortality in Europe, 1979–1993. Men and women, age 30 to 69 years.

In a well-recognized epidemiological concept the late Geoffrey Rose distinguished the determinants of sick individuals from those of sick populations [3]. He pointed out that to understand factors which determine incidence rates and prevalences of whole populations we need to study characteristics of whole populations, and not just of individuals. He contended that if populations are exposed to different environmental factors, to culturally determined life styles or diets, individual susceptibility or genetic predisposition cease to matter as determinants of disease rates as they can only modify the response to a generalized exposure of the population at large. To give an example, disease rates close to the Polar circle are different from those in the tropics, not because individuals are so drastically different but because the extrinsic factors are so predominant. Rose continued to claim that the characteristics of populations determine most of the occurrence of cardiovascular diseases.

Many physiological and life style risk factors have been investigated to assess this hypothesis. There were studies investigating population distributions of cholesterol or blood pressure levels, for example. They were able to identify major differences that exist between populations and confirmed that these differences operate in the same direction as the disease rates. Moreover, there is an extensive body of evidence showing that risk factors are also strong predictors of CVD occurrence within populations. It has to be noted further that the disease fractions attributed by risk factors are a function of the prevalence of risk factor categories and the associated relative risks [4]. The composition of these contributions in a complex multifactorial process such as atherosclerosis and CVD is difficult to disentangle. Therefore, care should be administered with claims that cardiovascular disease cannot be sufficiently explained by the established risk factors and that we need further factors to solve the puzzles.

What then about the role of infectious agents? I would like to relate the arguments to the epidemiologic dimensions of the CVD epidemic that I have tried to outline above. One point was that CVD rates rise with age. On the other hand, chlamydiae are known to cause a chronic persistent infection that starts early in life and that seems to parallel the development of atherosclerosis and cardiovascular disease. However, we have evidence only for a fairly strong association between the traditional risk factors and pathologically confirmed early lesions [5] and may thus infer that risk factors contribute already very early to the occurrence of preclinical CVD. Although it has been claimed during this conference that chlamydiae may be found in these lesions as well if we only searched thoroughly enough, the conclusive evidence is still missing.

How about the difference in disease rates between men and women? Androtropism is something that is well known in infectious diseases and it has also been forwarded as an argument in support of the infection hypothesis of CVD. However, is there scientific evidence confirming, for example, that the occurrence of infections with the incriminated agents differs in men and women to such an extent that it could plausibly explain why men get CVD more often, or why it is more persistent in men, or that it has a stronger affinity to the vascular walls in men than in women? Again, to my knowledge, there is no indication that this is actually the case.

Let us then turn to the magnitude of the disease rates and the differences between populations. In most populations high to very high seroprevalences of titers against, for example, *C. pneumoniae* or *H. pylori*, have been observed. In Japan, for instance, studies have shown that in densely populated areas there is exposure to Chlamydia very early in life and over 80 % of people in the older age groups show titers. On the other hand, ischemic heat disease rates are about the lowest in the world, and they are even declining. Likewise, CVD rates in many underdeveloped countries are at the bottom line of global CVD mortality rates while we know definitely that in particular in these regions of the world seroprevalences are high. I suppose that such inverse ecological associations contradict the hypothesis that infectious causes play a major role on the population level.

If we turn now to the CVD epidemic in Central and Eastern Europe with rises over the last decades we have to ask ourselves, are these trends due to unrecognized outbreaks of Chlamydia or other agents, or to particularly high infection rates and poor infection control or could it be that more virulent strains occur in this part of Europe? To me it appears difficult to conceive of any infectious process that would reasonably explain what is going on in these countries.

Finally, it has been proposed that the highly differential use and consumption of antibiotics in the world may be considered as a potential determinant differing between populations and over time. A very recent report from the US seems to support this hypothesis [6]. I would like to comment this study from a different, namely the population point of view. If one looks at the odds ratios of this study, there is indeed convincing statistical significance and strength of effects: taking quinolones was associated with a 55 % reduction of acute myocardial infarctions. But when one looks at the data from a population perspective, that is, at how frequently this drug was actually used, the quinolones were taken by only 8 out of

3,300 myocardial infarction cases and by 62 out of 14,000 controls. This is indeed very low and indicates that very, very few people in the population seem to take these antibiotics. Is this to explain plausibly trends in populations or in rate variations between populations? I doubt it strongly.

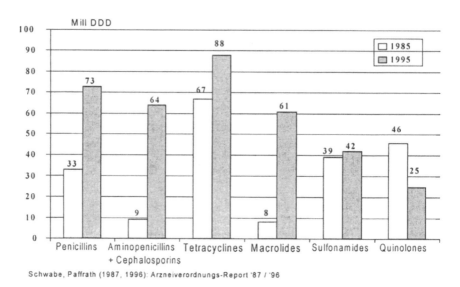

Figure 3. Prescriptions of antibiotics in Germany 1985 and 1995, in daily defined doses (DDD).

To expand on this, it has also been claimed that the decline in disease rates in the industrialized nations could be related to people taking generally more antibiotics. The next figure (Figure 3) was adapted from the *Arzneiverordnungsreport*, a German prescription report of drugs. The figure depicts millions of defined daily dosages (DDDs) of antibiotics used in 1985 and in 1995. It is true, there are strongly increasing rates in the numbers of DDDs prescribed in Germany. If we convert this, however, into numbers of patients taking antibiotics (in 1985 relative to a population of roughly 60 million, in 1995 after reunification roughly 80 million) we find that tetracyclines were taken at an amount of about one dose per head of the population per year. For others, like the macrolides or quinolones, the amounts were even less. This 'population dosage' cannot be seriously invoked to explain trends in CVD rates in the order of about 30 to 40 %.

I conclude that the infection hypothesis of atherosclerosis is novel, attractive, and scientifically challenging. It is plausible in a number of aspects and it is impressive with regard to some findings in atherosclerotic plaques. On the other hand, the evidence supporting the hypothesis is not consistent, in particular, when talking about population patterns and the epidemiologic dimensions of CVD. Presumably, there is a lot of publication bias: studies with positive results are being published more eagerly because they are controversial and attractive to the readership. They were probably also necessary to open up the field for discussion. It seems likely that negative studies are coming up only now. So we should be more patient and very careful to avoid an optimistic bias, that is, a selective evaluation or recognition of the scientific evidence. On the other hand, there is a strong background of evidence relating to the classical risk factors. From what has been presented in this symposium before, I do not see a great likelihood for infectious agents as primary causes of atherosclerosis. Moreover, I do not see that these agents are good candidates to explain the variations and trends of CVD in populations. Their precise role, if any, will have to be further elucidated and have to stand the test of time.

References

1. WHO MONICA Project (1989) Objectives and Design. Int J Epidemiol 18 (Supplement 2): 29–37
2. WHO MONICA Project (1994) Myocardial infarction and Coronary Deaths in the World Health Organization MONICA Project. Registration procedures, Event rates, and case-fatality rates in 38 populations from 21 countries in four continents. Circulation 90: 583–612
3. Rose G (1981) The strategy of prevention: lessons from cardiovascular disease. Br Med J 282: 1847–1851
4. Stamler J (1992) Established major coronary risk factors. In: Marmot M, Elliott P (eds) Coronary heart disease epidemiology – from aetiology to public health. Oxford Medical Publications
5. Strong JP, Malcolm GT, McMahan CA, Tracy RE, Newman WP, Hederick EE, Cornhill JF for the PDAY Research Group (1999) Prevalence and extent of atherosclerosis in adolescents and young adults. Implications for prevention from the Pathobiological Determinants of Atherosclerosis in Youth Studies. JAMA 281: 727–735
6. Meyer RM, Derby LE, Jick SS, Vasilakis C, Jick H (1999) Antibiotics and risk of subsequent first-time acute myocardial infarction. JAMA 281: 427–431

Discussion

Saikku:

I would like to comment this PDAY study because Kuo et al. in 1995 published a study where they showed that in 15-year-old boys in lipid plaques *C. pneumoniae* was more commonly found than in more advanced lesions.

Brade:

From the experimental work in infectious diseases in general we have learnt so much from experiments in animals and that the genetic background of the animals is tremendously important for the outcome of a disease. From the same species there are strains which are completely resistant towards certain microorganisms and others which are highly susceptible. Certainly the genetic background of individuals is also important in general for infectious diseases. Looking to putative attribution of infectious diseases to coronary heart disease from your epidemiological overview, do ethnic groups play any role in the distribution of the disease if you compare it with infections?

Hense:

First of all there are large differences between ethnic groups. There are certain clusters, for instance we know that the African-American population has certain characteristics that predispose them to stroke or renal disease, the South Asians have characteristics that seem to be genetically related to disorders close to the metabolic syndrome, and so on. Some people claim that also for the Asian populations the low lipid levels are related to different genetic backgrounds. But I don't see where the link is to the infectious diseases. To me the question is whether we have something like a necessary or a sufficient cause that is creating a disease. Where does the infectious agent come in in terms of explaining differences for instance between different ethnic groups?

Brade:

Or why the Finnish population should not have a different receptor for a certain microorganism than the rest of the European population.

Hense:

If there is any evidence to this end: perfect, that would be just the kind of evidence I would certainly consider valid. If you can prove it and if you show in addition that it has a high prevalence in the population, it may help to explain why this problem has been present in the Finnish population for a long time. To my knowledge, nothing has been identified that really makes the Finnish genetically very special. There are some clusters, some types, but there is no explanation in general of what is going on there. Another question is, why do we have such a drastic drop in rates? This is certainly not related or cannot be explained by genetic causes because such a drastic drop within 10, 15 years with the same genetic background is inexplicable to me.

Byrne:

We should start to consider things in terms of maybe "risky cohesion" rather than "risk factors", so that in the Asians you have one low known risk factor and then you impose an infection on top of that, because you need a certain risky cohesion to actually get disease in – you hinted at this when you said something about secondary causes playing a role, but it could be a primary cause with other risk factors. If we could devise a way to think of the proper risky cohesion where infectious agents, together with known risk factors, combine to contribute to the disease process in ways that make sense, this would be something worth thinking about.

Hense:

I couldn't agree more. We should go in this direction, this makes also for the attractiveness of the hypothesis. But the evidence there seems still very scarce.

Byrne:
But it is a new issue. We have been gathering evidence only for ten years.

Dunne:
You have shown the cardiovascular disease rates are dropping with time and you showed some distributions of cholesterol in Japan versus Finland and the distribution of blood pressures and how that causes the problem. Is there any data on the populations' transient mean cholesterol levels with time as well? You would want to see if those are the important risk factors themselves. You are going to see those dramatically dropping in order to help understand the shift other than just a point estimate.

Hense:
That is one of the questions that has been addressed by the MONICA project and that is under analysis right now. The publication is coming soon.

Dunne:
A US group's publication in *JAMA* about a year ago stated that they tried to assess that very question looking at shifts in those risk factors over time, the understanding being that we were using more cholesterol-lowering agents or that diet is better. It just was not strong enough. There were still a large fraction of risks that were not explained by shifts in those overall groups. At first you want to say, well, it explains it all, the cause of atherosclerosis is Chlamydia. I am not sure that we need to go there to explain all this. Maybe some of the risk factors are interacting, that is more important. If Ian said, the cholesterol was not important, hypertension is not important, they may be more important in the setting of infection or not. That is difficult to tease out in the early days of this whole kind of story.

Saikku:
I would like to comment this situation in Finland. We were the last industrialized country where *C. trachomatis* appeared. This susceptibility to chlamydial infections has not been thoroughly studied in Finland, but I think in North Sweden studies were done on HLA association with coronary heart disease.

Burger:
The proportion of non-infected or at least "not antibody-forming" persons in the population is roughly 2:3, both in males and females in all countries. Did anybody ever look in the non-infected part of this population? Are there common factors which might explain a particular resistance or genetic elements? Not risk factors in the infected ones, but what is the reason for resistance?

Hense:
Or what protects people from getting infected? I don't know.

Byrne:

Just because someone does not have an antibody response does not mean they are not infected. They could be infected and not making response, and in fact those people may be more at risk, for all we know.

4.2
The epidemiology of *Chlamydia pneumoniae* versus the epidemiology of potential Chlamydial diseases (Atherosclerosis, Multiple Sclerosis, M. Alzheimer)

W. Stille, C. Stephan, M. Madeo, E. Bauer-Krylov

Chronic infection with *Chlamydia pneumoniae* has been associated with:

- Sarcoidosis
- Asthma
- Atherosclerosis
- Erythema nodosum
- Endocarditis
- Myocarditis
- Thyroiditis
- Arthritis
- Encephalitis
- Multiple Sclerosis
- Guillain-Barré syndrome
- M. Alzheimer
- Lung cancer
- Essential hypertension

Both the incidence of infection with *Chlamydia pneumoniae* and the incidence of the different diseases follow different patterns. The comparison of the epidemiology of infection with *Chlamydia pneumoniae* with the epidemiology of certain other diseases, e.g. atherosclerosis, multiple sclerosis and Alzheimer's disease, seems to attract some interest.

Epidemiology of *Chlamydia pneumoniae*

The transmission of *Chlamydia pneumoniae* happens by human-to-human contact. It is apparently not highly infectious. Usually infection takes place due to a relatively close contact. Family outbreaks are common. Obviously there is no animal reservoir. Infections may have an endemic or epidemic cause with waves every 7 years. There is no protective immunity; every person gets several infections during life. There can be a high percentage of long-term carriers, mainly in day-care facilities.

Seroepidemiology

Last decade's investigations show a high prevalence of antibodies against *Chlamydia pneumoniae* in all populations around the world. Obviously there are no marked differences in different ethnic groups (Figure 1).

Generally speaking, infections with *Chlamydia pneumoniae* are uncommon below the age of 5 years in developed countries [8], with the exception of children attending day-care centers [9]. Antibody titers increase permanently during childhood within years. Males have more and higher antibodies. However, serology is not reliable; infection may be possible despite the lack of antibodies [10]. The patients may have a high incidence of immune-complexes in blood. The age-dependent increase in detection was also reported in a study of 59 heart transplant donors [11]. PCR was positive in 13 of 59 healthy donors. There were no positive reactions in 23 donors below 15 years, but 4 of 5 donors at age 15 were positive. Apparently primary infections of the vascular tissue by *Chlamydia pneumoniae* mainly takes place at the age between 10 and 20.

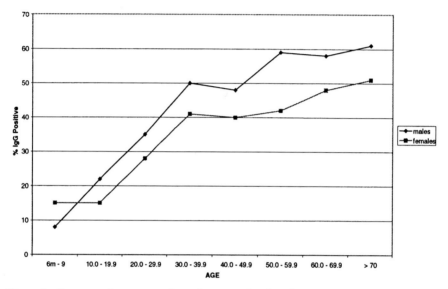

Figure 1. *C. pneumoniae* seroprevalence in a sample of an immunocompetent population in Milan, Italy

The epidemiology of atherosclerosis is quite different from the epidemiology of acute chlamydial infections. There are marked differences in the incidences of coronary heart disease worldwide (Figure 2).

The MONICA Project results compare incidences of worldwide cardiovascular disease. In the MONICA Project the lowest incidence of myocardial infarction was found in China. Finland and the northern parts of the U.K. had the highest incidences. There is a marked over-mortality in coronary infarction in male patients aged 34–64. This over-mortality could not be found in China. Concerning official data on cardiovascular disease by the WHO, there are slightly different incidences. Certain parts of the former Soviet Union take a leading position. Germany is in the upper center. The lowest incidence in Europe is in Albania, but the lowest incidence worldwide was registered in sub-Saharan African states like Zimbabwe or in South Korea.

Onset of Atherosclerosis apparently is in youth. The first data results primarily from victims of the Korea war [2]. In the so-called PDAY study the atherosclerosis in younger Americans was evaluated [1]. Fatty streaks as the first tissue changes in atherosclerosis can be seen at the age of 15–19 years. Further on, there is an advancement of lesions from 15 to 34 years. No marked differences were found either between black and white Americans, or between females and males. – This is in contrast to the general sex relation of atherosclerotic diseases compared males versus females. There is a 7 times higher incidence of coronary heart disease at the age between 35 and 44 in males. In recent decades the mortality of atherosclerosis was not observed as stable. There has been a marked decline of atherosclerosis and its mortality in western countries since 1970. The decline is far more pronounced in the United States than it is in England, Wales, Scotland and Finland. One possible explanation could be seen in the antibiotic policy – the U.K. and Finland have a quite restrictive antibiotic policy (Figure 3).

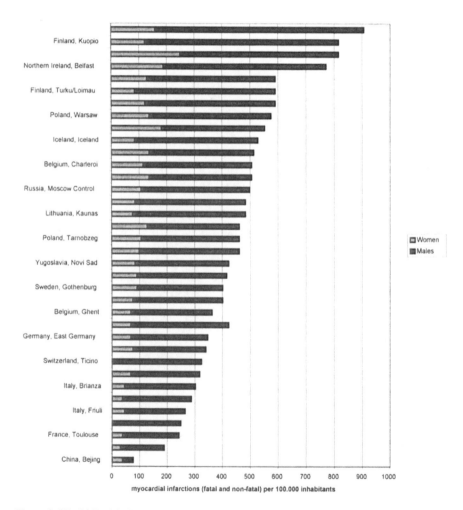

Figure 2. World Health Organization / MONICA-Project: comparison of myocardial infarctions per 100,000 in 35 to 64-year-old population (basic data 1985–87), age-adjusted annual rates for males and women of all study centers.

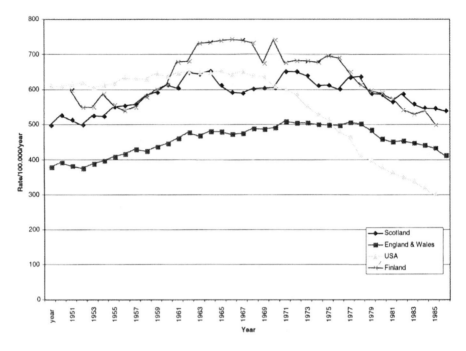

Figure 3. Trends in CHD mortality in four countries during the period 1950–87: annual rate per 100,000 men aged 40–69. Age-standardized rates from WHO

The decrease of mortality of coronary infarction is present also in Germany [12]. The decrease started in different years, in different age groups. There are various possible explanations for the decrease of the incidence of coronary disease since the period between 1965 and 1970. From the conventional point of view, better lifestyle (diet, smoking, weight) and better treatment (cardiac diseases, hypertension) are used as an explanation. From the infectiologist's viewpoint the popularization of antibiotics since 1965 must be regarded as a major argument [13].

The protective effect of prior antibiotic use was shown by a prominent American group [14]. An analysis of data of the National Health Service in the U.K. compares patients with acute major myocardial infarctions with matched controls. There was a significant protective effect of prior antibiotic use, namely tetracyclines and chinolones, in preventing the development of myocardial infarction. Concerning macrolides, no differences were shown, however the primary substance used was erythromycin with no sufficient activity against Chlamydia.

Antibiotics can also be regarded as explanation of the so-called "French paradox": The incidence of coronary infarction in France is only 50 % of that in its neighbor Germany. The usual explanation is the large consumption of cheap red wine containing many antioxidants. Another explanation is the much more popularized consumption of antichlamydial antibiotics in France, i.e. modern macrolides and tetracyclines.

In medical text books the pathogenesis of atherosclerosis is often explained as a "response to injury". Different risk factors and vascular micro-trauma lead to typical involvement of the major arteries. The response-to-injury theory was first defined by Russell Ross 1976 [3] and was updated several times. The last remarkable revision was in January 1999 by Ross [4]. Atherosclerosis now becomes an "inflammatory disease". Thus there was a remarkable change in the interpretation of the pathogenesis of atherosclerosis within the last 25 years.

There have been several weak aspects in traditional explanations of atherogenesis. Atherosclerosis apparently is not a storage disease of lipids. Atheroma do *not* contain large amounts of lipids (3–5 %). Atheroma are usually free of oxidized lipoproteins. Atheroma consist mainly of necrotic protein. The amount of calcium may be much higher than the amount of cholesterol. So atherogenesis can be evaluated as a chronic inflammation followed by secondary lipoidosis and secondary calcification.

There are geographical arguments against the risk factor concept of atherosclerosis: Smoking is not a confounding risk factor of atherosclerosis in Korea and Mexico. Hypertension does not lead to atherosclerosis in sub-Saharan Africans (but in Afro-Americans). Diabetes does not lead to atherosclerois in certain aborigine peoples (Pima, Nauru/Australia). In certain countries with very low incidence of atherosclerosis like Thailand, people have the same amount of cholesterol in adolescence as in Germany.

The risk factor concept should be viewed with general caution. Risk factors may be valid only if patients suffer from chronic chlamydial endarteritis. Certain "risk factors" can be evaluated as epiphenomenon of chronic smoldering infection, e.g. elevated CRP and fibrinogen. The so-called "atherogenic dyslipidemia" in atherosclerosis patients may be a characteristic of chronic persisting chlamydial infection and not a risk factor.

As a conclusion, the interpretation of atherosclerosis as ultrachronic smoldering chlamydial infection of the arteries is much better founded than the actual explanation of atherosclerosis as the consequence of heterogeneous risk factors.

Epidemiology of Multiple Sclerosis

Multiple sclerosis follows a geographical distribution similar to atherosclerosis. In general, countries with high incidences of atherosclerosis also do have high prevalences of multiple sclerosis.

Multiple sclerosis is a disease with an uneven gender relation of female to male, that is 2 : 1. Typically MS is a disease of younger females at the age of 15–40, onset after the age of 40 is rare. Persons with higher social level are more often affected. There are obscure reports of a few clusters of diseases.

Despite the improved diagnostics, there seems to be a general tendency of stagnation, respectively a decrease in prevalence during the recent decades. Migrants usually keep the risk of their home country at the age of adolescence in regard to a development of MS. It was not possible to find reliable data on the epidemiology of multiple sclerosis in the tropics.

An established risk factor of multiple sclerosis is the higher incidence of respiratory infections in childhood and adolescence. Histologically there are certain similarities of atherosclerosis and multiple sclerosis. In the tissues of both diseases there are foam cell formations, inflammatory cells and inflammatory mediators. The demyelinization in multiple sclerosis can be evaluated as a focal change of lipid metabolism. As epidemiological observation, *Chlamydia pneumoniae* fulfills perfectly the requirements of the potential agents of multiple sclerosis, postulated by Kurtzke in the Faroer analysis [5]. As a conclusion, common intravascular infection by Chlamydia should have local consequences in vessel's surrounding tissue. Maybe the plaques of multiple sclerosis are metastatic foci of exacerbated smoldering vascular infection by *Chlamydia pneumoniae*.

Epidemiology of Alzheimer's Disease

Alzheimer's disease also is very common in modern western societies. Up to 2 % of the general population may suffer from Alzheimer's disease. There is a remarkable increase in high age that may lead to very high percentages of patients above 80 years. Analyzing senile dementia in the tropics, apparently Alzheimer's disease is rare to very rare there, may be even non-existing [7]. There is only one clinical study that compares prevalences of Alzheimer's disease in a Nigerian (Ibadan) with an US-American (Indianapolis) community, finding a significant lower prevalence of clinical Alzheimer's in Nigeria [15]. A potential connection with Chlamydia infection is, up to now, only one *post mortem* study [6].

Conclusion

An interpretation of different diseases' pathogenesis is difficult. May be the key issue of the pathogenesis is the age of primary infection with the pathogen *Chlamydia pneumoniae*. Early infection in childhood may lead to certain protection of generalized consequences later on. This would be analogous to other infections' pathogenesis. Later onset of infection leads to more severe diseases, e.g. vascular involvement ("yet an other poliomyelitis story"). As a consequence of the very common vascular involvement usually known as atherosclerosis, in a small percentage of patients metastatic plaques in brain arise. This is a disease we usually call multiple sclerosis. Thus multiple sclerosis would be a relatively rare localized metastatic consequence of the central nervous system (CNS), originating from a chronic smoldering vascular infection by Chlamydia. According to this theory, in higher ages the CNS loses the capability to localize the infectious processes caused by *Chlamydia pneumoniae*. A possible result could be a generalized brain involvement – the common late idiopathic form of Alzheimer's disease.

Though step by step we are getting a clearer image of what *Chlamydia pneumoniae* infection is and could be, the complete pathology of this pathogen still remains cryptic. In German there is a proverb: "There is still much to be done. Let's get started!" – *Es gibt viel zu tun – packen wir's an!*

References

1. Strong JP, Malcom GT, McMahan CA, Tracy RE, Newman WP, Herderick EE, Cornhill JF (1999) Prevalence and Extent of Atherosclerosis in Adolescents and Young Adults. JAMA 281 (8): 727–735
2. Enos WF, Holmes RH, Beyer J (1953) Coronary disease among United States soldiers killed in action in Korea. JAMA 152: 1090–1093
3. Ross R, Glomset JA (1976) The pathogenesis of atherosclerosis. N Engl J Med 295 (7): 369–377
4. Ross R (1999) Atherosclerosis – An inflammatory disease. N Engl J Med 340 (2): 115–126
5. Kurtzke JF, Hyllested K, Heltberg A (1993) Multiple Sclerosis in the Faroes. In: Firnhaber W, Lauer K (eds) Multiple Sclerosis in Europe. Leuchtturm-Verlag/LTV Press, Alsbach/Bergstraße
6. Balin BJ, Gerard HC, Arking EJ, Appelt DM, Branigan PJ, Abrams JT, Whittum-Hudson JA, Hudson AP (1998) Identification and localization of *Chlamydia pneumoniae* in the Alzheimer's brain. Med Microbiol Immunol 187 (1): 23–42
7. Jorm AF (1990) The epidemiology of Alzheimer's disease and related disorders. Chapman and Hall, London
8. Blasi F, Cosentini R, Schoeller MC, Lupo A, Allegra L (1993) *Chlamydia pneumoniae* seroprevalence in immunocompetent and immunocompromised populations in Milan. Thorax 48: 1261–1263
9. Normann E, Gnarpe J, Gnarpe H, Wettergren B (1998) *Chlamydia pneumoniae* in children attending day-care centers in Gävle, Sweden. Pediatr Infect Dis J 17 (6): 474–478
10. Maass M, Bartels C, Kruger S, Krause E, Engel PM, Dalhoff K (1998) Endovascular presence of *Chlamydia pneumoniae* DNA is a generalized phenomenon in atherosclerotic vascular disease. Atherosclerosis 140 Suppl 1: S25–S30
11. Taylor-Robinson D, Ong G, Thomas BJ, Rose ML, Yacoub MH (1998) *Chlamydia pneumoniae* in vascular tissues from heart-transplant donors. Lancet 351 (9111): 1255
12. Willich S, Löwel H, Mey W, Trautner C (1999) Regionale Unterschiede der Herz-Kreislauf-Mortalität in Deutschland. Dt Ärztebl 96: A-483–488
13. Ånestad G, Scheel O, Hungnes O (1997) Chronic infections and coronary heart disease. Lancet 350: 1028
14. Meier CR, Derby LE, Jick SS, Vasilakis C, Jick H (1999) Antibiotics and risk of subsequent first-time acute myocardial infarction. JAMA 281 (5): 427–431
15. Hall K, Gureje O, Gao S, Ogunniyi A, Hui SL, Baiyewu O, Unverzagt FW, Oluwole S, Hendrie HC (1998) Risk factors and Alzheimer's disease: a comparative study of two communities. Aust N Z J Psychiatry 32 (5): 698–706
16. United Nations (1996) Demographic Yearbook 1994, New York
17. Lauer K (1993) Epidemiologie der multiplen Sklerose. In: Henkes H, Kölmel HW (eds) Die entzündlichen Erkrankungen des Zentralnervensystems: Handbuch und Atlas. (3. Ergänzungslieferung 2/1997). Ecomed, Landsberg/Lech

Discussion

Bhakdi:
I can't respond to all the things I disagree on because of time constraints.

Stille:
As usual.

Bhakdi:
Because I do come from Thailand I must say that this sort of statistics is very screwed. It depends where in Thailand you measure your cholesterol. In Bangkok with the rich people we measure the same cholesterol that you have, but if you go to the Northeast of Thailand, you have very low cholesterol. When we look at the values that you showed, 160, 170 total cholesterol, that is low. This is not the value we have here. In fact, in Northeast Thailand we do have values around 150 to 170 cholesterol. But about one third of that is HDL, and it is only the LDL that is atherogenic, as we know. When looking at these statistics, let us be fair about it.

Stille:
Let us be fair at the other side. There can be no doubt, atherosclerosis is extremely rare in a country like Thailand and there are other comparable countries, too, and it is a disease of Western society, Western lifestyle.

Bhakdi:
What I am trying to say is that it is rare with us because we have very little LDL cholesterol which is the major risk factor of atherosclerosis. If you go through all those statistics and ask, what is the major risk factor that downs the statistics, you will find that it is the LDL cholesterol and the HDL cholesterol, and this is accepted. We have to discuss this in the context of a general knowledge of risk factors, and it is not correct to say that the atheroma does not contain lipid. There are atheromas full of free cholesterol which is typical of atherosclerosis, it does not occur with syphilis, it does not occur with tuberculosis, it is typical for the atheroma.

Stille:
No.

Bhakdi:
Of course the phospholipids can be taken away, but not the free cholesterol. And that is what drives its formation.

Stille:
The content of an atheroma is protein and not lipid.

4.3
The high male mortality of coronary heart diseases can be explained as a result of chronic infection

E. Bauer-Krylov, W. Stille

The higher incidence of coronary infarction in younger males (age 35 to 60) is well known but difficult to explain.

In the years 1990 to 1997 in Germany the general statistical relation male to female in ischaemic heart diseases is 1:1.06 (Figure 1). The overmortality at younger age in males is 1:5 [1]. The male overmortality is also present in all the other western countries; this phenomenon is difficult to explain.

The traditional explanations are male behavior, testosterone and higher lipids. Men are in their behavior work-orientated, involved in aggressive and competitive roles and ambitious. They develop more than females the "Coronary Prone Behavior Pattern" [2]. Testosterone makes men aggressive and supports their behavior. Males have slightly higher lipids than females which is explained by the estrogens which increase the HDL and decrease the LDL [3].

Chronic persisting arteriitis by *Chlamydia pneumoniae* can be due a new explanation for the pathogenesis of atherosclerosis ("Atherosclerosis is the trachoma of the aorta"). If we regard atherosclerosis as chronic smoldering bacterial infection, an uneven sex distribution is not unique. Infectious diseases have a marked male overmortality at younger age (Figure 2).

The similarity of the age and sex distribution of all infectious diseases (without HIV) compared with ischaemic heart diseases is impressive. The distribution follows the same type.

Many bacterial infections have a much higher incidence in males. The well-known fact that lobar pneumonia is a disease of younger men can also be seen in this graph (Figure 3). We found a similar distribution in septicaemia (Figure 4). Also bacterial meningitis shows a similar distribution (Figure 5). In tuberculosis the male overmortality is very marked (Figure 6); it is present in all age groups.

Even appendicitis as a bacterial disease with mixed pathogens shows the overmortality of males at younger age (Figure 7).

In 1992 H.E. Müller from Braunschweig emphasized the stronger female resistance to infectious diseases (Table 1) [4]. He showed that females have a higher resistance to most infectious agents. The stronger female resistance was explained by the females' sex hormones, especially the estrogens.

Potential explanations for the better protection of females are:

1. Females have a very complicated parturition and need a better protection against infectious complications.
2. The protection disappears with the climacteric period.
3. Estrogen substitution protects against coronary heart disease but also against infections.

4. Female animals are better protected against bacterial infection [5].
5. The higher life expectancy of female mice is not present in germ-free conditions [6].
6. Estrogen stimulates humoral immunity and cell-mediated response [7].
7. Females have higher immunglobulin levels than men due to the sex hormones [8] and due to the X-chromosome [9].

The male overmortality by coronary heart disease could not be explained by the actual theory of the pathogenesis of atherosclerosis as the summary of different risk factors over years ("response-to-injury theory"). But male overmortality is easy to explain if we regard atherosclerosis as a result of a chronic smoldering chlamydial infection.

References

1. Statistisches Bundesamt (1997) Todesursachen in Deutschland 1990 bis 1997. Fachserie 12 Gesundheitswesen (Reihe 4). Statistisches Bundesamt, Wiesbaden
2. Waldron I (1976) Why do women live longer than men? Soc Sci Med 10: 349–362
3. Barrett-Connor E, Bush T (1989) Estrogen replacement and coronary heart disease. Cardiovasc Clin 19 (3): 159–172
4. Müller HE (1992) Das leistungsfähigere Abwehrsystem der Frau gegen Infektionen. Wiener Med Wochenschr 42: 389–395
5. Goble FC, Konopka EA (1973) Sex as a factor in infectious diseases. Trans NY Acad Sci 35: 325–346
6. Gordon HA, Bruckner-Kardoss E, Wostmann BS (1966) Aging in germ-free mice: life tables and lesions observed at natural death. J Gerontol 21: 380–387
7. Schuurs AH, Verheul HA (1990) Effects of gender and sex steroids on the immune response. J Steroid Biochem 35: 157–172
8. Ahmed SA, Penhale WJ, Talal N (1985) Sex hormones, immune response and autoimmune diseases. Am J Path 121: 531–551
9. Rhodes K, Markham RL, Maxwell PM, Monk-Jones ME (1969) Immunglobulins and the X-Chromosome. BMJ 3: 439–441

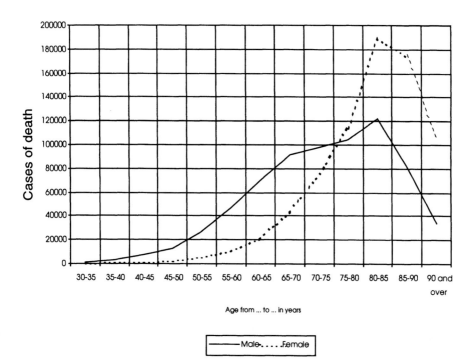

Figure 1. Cases of death in Germany for ischaemic heart diseases (ICD 410–414) from 1990 to 1997 by sex and age (n=1,441,358), Statistisches Bundesamt [1].

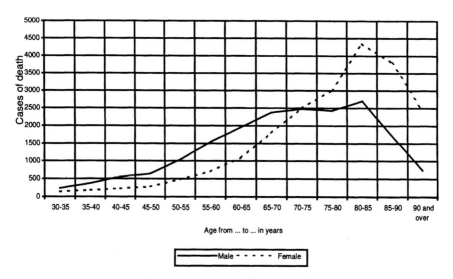

Figure 2. Cases of death in Germany for infectious diseases (ICD 001–139) without HIV (ICD 042–044) from 1990 to 1997 (n=39,773), Statistisches Bundesamt [1].

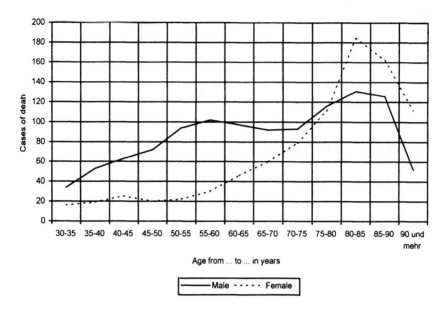

Figure 3. Cases of death in Germany for pneumococcal pneumonia (ICD 481) from 1990 to 1997 by sex and age (n=2,012), Statistisches Bundesamt [1].

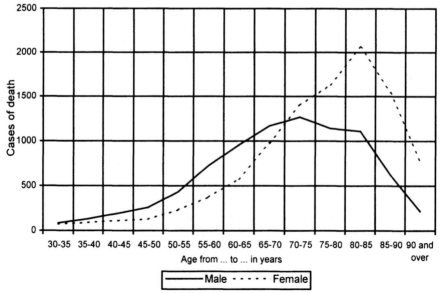

Figure 4. Cases of death in Germany for septicaemia (ICD 038) from 1990 to 1997 by sex and age (n=18,271), Statistisches Bundesamt [1].

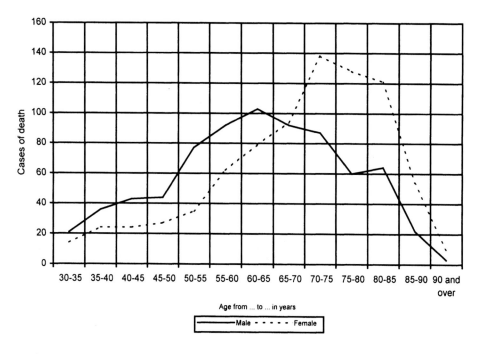

Figure 5. Cases of death in Germany for bacterial meningitis (ICD 320) from 1990 to 1997 by sex and age (n=1,554), Statistisches Bundesamt [1].

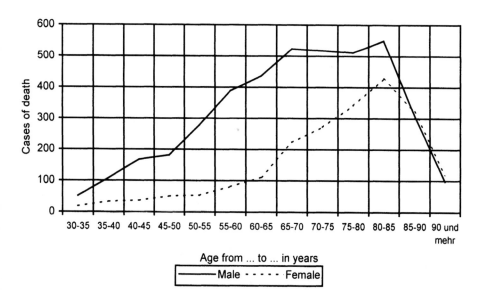

Figure 6. Cases of death in Germany for tuberculosis (ICD 010–018) from 1990 to 1997 by sex and age (n=6,211), Statistisches Bundesamt [1].

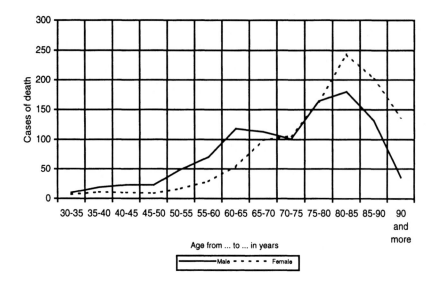

Figure 7. Cases of death in Germany for appendicitis (ICD 540–543) from 1990 to 1997 by sex and age (n=2,125), Statistisches Bundesamt [1].

Table 1. The sex ratio male-to-female (m:f) in bacteria-caused clinical syndrome (signed with *: a sex-related exposure is discussed) (by H.E.Müller [4]).

Actinomyces israelii	Actinomycosis	80:20	Lerner	1973
		75:25	Weese et al.	1975
Afipia felis	Cat scratch disease, loc. infection	57:43	Margileth et al.	1987
	Systemic disease	70:30	Margileth et al.	1987
Bartonella bacilliformis	Oroya-Fever	71:29	Gray et al.	1990
Campylobacter fetus	Bacteraemia	78:22	Stille et al.	1969
		64:36	Ullmann	1975
C. intestinalis	Bacteraemia	63:37	Guerrant et al.	1978
C. jejuni	Bacteraemia	60:40	Guerrant et al.	1978
Clostridium perfringens	Enteritis necroticans	64:36	Schoop	1969
Corynebacterium diphtheriae	Diphtheria	75:25	Gross et al.	1978
Enterococcus spec.	Meningitis	65:35	Buchs	1977
Erysipelothrix rhusiopathiae	Endocarditis, sepsis	89:11	Volmer et al.	1976
Escherichia coli O157	Haemolytic anemia in children	08:92	Rowe et al.	1991
Haemophilus ducreyi	Ulcus molle	90-95: 5-10	Braun-Falco et al.	1978
Haemophilus influenzae	Pneumonia with bacteremia	57:43	Wallace et al.	1978
	Pneumonia without bacteremia	83:17	Wallace et al.	1978
Legionella pneumophila	Legionnaires disease, sporadic	71:29	Anonymus	1978
	" in small epidemic area	74:26	Anonymus	1978
Listeria monocytogenes	Septicemia	69:39	Kampelmacher et al.	1980
	Meningitis	83:17	Kampelmacher et al.	1980

Organism	Condition	Ratio	Author	Year
Mycobacterium tuberculosis	Pulmonary tuberculosis	75:25	Anonymus	1977
		63:37	Muhar et al.	1978
	Active Pulmonary Tuberculosis	74:26	Popp	1971
	Inactive Pulmonary Tuberculosis	60:40	Popp	1971
Mycobacterium avium	Pulmonary mycobacteriosis	69:04	Schröder	1977
	Mycobacteriosis	55:45	O'Brien et al.	1987
Mycobacterium avium/ Intracellulare	Mycobacteriosis	66:34	Ahn et al.	1979
		75-80: 25-20	Rosenzweig et al.	1981
Mycobacterium kansasii	Pulm. mycobacteriosis	100:0	Schröder	1977
	Mycobacteriosis	73:27	Ahn et al.	1979
Mycobacterium spec.=	Pulm. mycobacteriosis	75-80: 25-20	Schröder	1977
("atypic mycobacteria")	Cervical gland – mycobacteriosis	55:45	Schröder	1977
		75:25	Lincoln et al.	1972
	Mycobacteriosis	59:41	O'Brien	1987
Neisseria meningitidis	Asymptomatic colonization	60:40	Cartwright et al.	1987
	Meningitis	60:40	Weise	1976
Salmonella spec.	Salmonellosis, all	50,3:49,7	Anonymus	1977
	Salmonellosis in adolescent < 20 yr	54:46	Anonymus	1977
	Salmonellosis in adult > 20 yr	44:56*	Anonymus	1977
Serratia marcescens	Bacteraemia	75:25	v. Graevenitz et al.	1980
	Arthritis	67:33	v. Graevenitz et al.	1980
Streptococcus pyogenes	Pharyngitis in adult	53:47	Chretien et al.	1979
Strept.coccus agalactiae	Pharyngitis in adult	43:57*	Chretien et al.	1979
	Asymptomatic colonization In neonate	57:43	Baker et al.	1973
	Neonatal infection, all	64:36	Wilkinson et al.	1973
		69:31	Cayeux	1972
	"Early Onset"- Septicemia	57:43	Reid	1975
	"Late Onset"- Meningitis	69:31	Reid	1975
		53:47	Quirante et at.	1974
		53:47	Franciosi et al.	1973
		52:48	Baker et al.	1974
		45:55	Baker at al.	1973
		18:82	Barton et al.	1973
Treponema pallidum	Benign Lues III	47:53	Brunsgaard et al.	1955
	Cardiovascular Lues III	65:35	Brunsgaard et al.	1955
	Neuro-Lues (Lues IV)	35:35	Brunsgaard et al.	1955
Vibrio cholerae	Cholera	53:47	Velimirovic et al.	1974
Yersinia enterocolitica	Yersiniosis	60:40	Baier et al.	1979
		56:44	Bockemühl et al.	1978
Yersinia pestis	Plague mortality, all	75:25	Burnet	1971
		83:17	Ell	1984
	" " young adult	67:33	Ell	1984
	" " adolescent >15J	69:31	Ell	1984
	" " adolescent <15J	50:50	Ell	1984

4.4
The *Spandauer Gesundheitstest* – Retrospective cohort study on *Chlamydia pneumoniae* infections and cardiovascular disease – A study concept

T. Ziese

Introduction

There is rising epidemiological evidence on the association of *Chlamydia pneumoniae* infections and cardiovascular diseases available [1], indicating major public health intervention possibilities. However, most of this evidence is derived from case control studies [1]. Case control studies are more prone to biases such as selection bias and recall bias than cohort studies. Moreover cohort studies provide better information on the temporal associations of different risks and diseases. Up to now only 4 studies with cohort design have been published [2, 3, 4, 5]. The Robert Koch-Institut considers to conduct a retrospective cohort study using a population which has now been under surveillance for almost 20 years.

Study goals

This proposed study shall cover the following main objectives:
- to describe the association between *Chlamydia pneumoniae* infections and cardiovascular disease over a period of 18 years,
- to describe the temporal relationship and the interaction between 'classical' cardiovascular risk factors and Chlamydia infections over time,
- to identify, to describe and to compare sub-populations with and without Chlamydia infections at increased risk for cardiovascular events later in life,
- to identify predictors for cardiovascular events in relation to the *Chlamydia pneumoniae*-antibody status for public health intervention strategies.

Study outline

We suggest to perform a retrospective cohort study with a population consisting of a group of exposed test persons with positive *Chlamydia pneumoniae* serology (cases) and a group of non-exposed test persons (controls) who all initially are free of cardiovascular diseases. The outcome variable is the occurrence of any cardiovascular event (death or disease).

Since 1982 every two years a study population of 6,700 persons has been monitored in Spandau, a district of Berlin. The monitoring included an examination part (height, weight, blood pressure), blood specimen and a questionnaire covering information on cardiovascular risk factors (socio-economic status, smoking, nutrition, alcohol consumption, physical activity, health care utilization), morbidity (hypertension, angina pectoris, myocardial infarction, stroke, chronic bronchitis, self-perceived health etc). Data also exist on height, weight, lung function, and blood pressure. *Chlamydia pneumoniae* serostatus, cholesterol levels and other parameters relevant for cardiovascular diseases can be determined from the blood specimens taken throughout the study time.

Information on five different examination waves is available for 1,800 participants (resp. 1,000 for eight cycles). The study is still ongoing. About 1,000 study participants died during the study period, the information on the cause of death is available for half of the cases yet.

The following steps have to be made:
- determination of the *Chlamydia pneumoniae* serostatus in the cohort,
- follow-up of cohort losses,
- setting up an appropriate dataset,
- statistical modeling and analysis.

Ad 1. Determination of the Chlamydia pneumoniae *serostatus in the cohort*

The basic concept of the planned study is to observe and analyze the occurrence of cardiovascular diseases within the study population in relation to the initial status of *Chlamydia pneumoniae* infection.

The first serum sample each, taken from those of the 1,800 study participants having taken part in at least five consecutive tests, shall be selected for serology of *Chlamydia pneumoniae*. For the matter of minimizing costs, additional investigations will be restricted to comparing the last serum samples taken from late participants with their initial samples, in order to detect any seroconversions.

The methods for defining past or ongoing infections with *Chlamydia pneumoniae*, especially by serology, is still a major problem [6]. As the amount of stored serum is very limited, we decided to postpone this step until a generally accepted and standardized method of *Chlamydia pneumoniae* serology has been established.

Ad 2. Follow-up of cohort losses

In the course of the long observation period, approximately 1,000 participants of the cohort have died. The latest survey of causes of death was performed in 1996 and should be up-dated in the frame of this project. Presently, the cause of death is unknown for 400 persons. In addition to death certificates, the cause of death is confirmed by medical records if available to improve reliability.

Ad 3. Data set

So far, the "*Spandauer Gesundheitstest*" has been used mainly for performing cross-sectional analyses, therefore not all of the available data is in a format for time series analyses yet. Integration of data from the current examination wave, linkage of the participants of different study periods, correction, and internal plausibility checks have been started.

Ad 4. Modeling and analysis

The statistical models are applied with the outcome parameter being "cardiovascular event" (illness or death). The following aspects shall be covered:
- Description of the relation between the occurrence of a *Chlamydia pneumoniae* infection and a later cardiovascular disease (procedure: Risk estimation using the logistic regression, Cox Proportional Hazard)
- Identification, description, and comparison of test groups with or without a Chlamydia infection, developing a cardiovascular disease in the course of the study (procedure: Variance analysis)
- Identification of predictors for future cardiovascular diseases in relation to *Chlamydia pneumoniae* infection. By means of these predictors, persons can be identified who are at higher risk for cardiovascular diseases and should therefore be targeted by prevention strategies (procedure: Logistic regression, Cox Proportional Hazard).

References

1. Danesh J, Collins R, Peto R (1997) Chronic infections and coronary heart disease: is there a link? Lancet 350: 430–436
2. David P, Strachan DP, Carrington D, Mendall MA (1999) Relation of *Chlamydia pneumoniae* serology to mortality and incidence of ischaemic heart disease over 13 years in the Caerphilly prospective heart disease study. BMJ 318: 1035–1040
3. Saikku P, Leinonen M, Tenkanen L, Linnanmaki E, Ekman MR, Manninen V, et al. (1992) Chronic *Chlamydia pneumoniae* infection as a risk factor for coronary heart disease in the Helsinki heart study. Ann Intern Med 116: 273–278
4. Ossewaarde JM, Feskens EJM, de Vries A, Vallinga CE, Kromhout D (1998) *Chlamydia pneumoniae* is a risk factor for coronary heart disease in symptom-free elderly men, but *Helicobacter pylori* and cytomegalovirus are not. Epidemiol Infect 120: 93–99
5. Miettinen H, Lehto S, Saikku P, Haffner SM, Rönnemaa T, Pyörälä K, et al. (1996) Association of *Chlamydia pneumoniae* and acute coronary heart disease events in non-insulin dependent diabetic and non-diabetic subjects in Finland. Eur Heart J 17: 682–688
6. Wang SP, Grayston JT (1984) Microimmunofluorescence serology in *Chlamydia trachomatis*. In: de la Maza LM, Peterson EM (eds) International Symposium on Medical Virology. Medical virology III: proceedings of the 1983 International Symposium on Medical Virology, held on October 19–21, 1983, in Anaheim, California, U.S.A. Elsevier, New York

Discussion

Brade:
Concerning the last transparency where you said it is quite easy to look to a group of people which have been treated for Helicobacter to see what is changing with regard to the reactivity towards pneumonia, I think one should include people

with tuberculosis which have been treated with Rifampicin. Rifa is the most active drug against Chlamydia. I think, perhaps you can learn from this group something as well.

Ziese:

I doubt if we have them in the study population, these are typical middle-class people, not the population you expect to have tuberculosis.

Hense:

Are there any comments with regard to the type of the set-up of the study, that is, the serological approach, the antibody approach, whether this is still appropriate? We heard that the antibodies are not very informative. Does it make sense with 80 % having high titers in that age group?

Stille:

I am a little bit against new serological studies. If you find a correlation, what are the consequences? It is already known. Or you find no correlation, then we have to put the serological procedure into question marks. At least, serology in Germany is not done in the optimal way. Only very few institutions make micro-immune fluorescence, they work with certain commercial reagents and the data is mainly a waste of money.

Ziese:

You are right concerning the reliability of antibody testing but there is nothing else available.

Stille:

That's no argument.

Ziese:

Most of the evidence we have so far, that there is an association between Chlamydia and cardiovascular diseases at all, is based on seroepidemiological evidence. Compare this to the situation concerning Helicobacter a couple of years ago. There were some studies indicating there is an association, but they were lacking the adjustment for confounders, not taking into account the whole system which leads to atherosclerosis. Then over time those studies have been published, and an association between Helicobacter and atherosclerosis is now hardly discussed any more or has even been denied by Peto in the *Lancet* in August 1997. A second argument in favor of doing the study is that it is the first time we can consider a long-time period, which has not been done before.

Brade:

We should not put serology in this negative aspect at present. We know so little about serology. The contribution by Gunna Christiansen showed in a very nice way how little we understand about the immuno-reactivity of different components of Chlamydia. We are at present only looking to those which are appearing on gels.

Maybe we have never seen the most relevant antigens as a band on a gel. To collect the material and have it ready for the time when the appropriate serological assays will have been established, can be very helpful. At present I agree that there is no other chance than doing it by the micro-immuno-fluorescence assay.

Anonymus:

What would be the best material to collect for the time being? Is that cells, white cells, is it DNA? Buffy coat?

Brade:

I would say serum because after all what we have heard already I am not convinced that a PCR protocol will be the parameter which makes the decision for either treating or not treating someone who is at risk. The serological parameters which we have at present certainly cannot help you. We have seen that 60 % are positive. But I am convinced that one day, if we get support to do all the work which should have been done during the last 20 years (the chlamydiologists have known the question for more than 20 years but we have not been supported to do this work appropriately), then we could provide you within perhaps five years with what are relevant antigens within *C. pneumoniae*.

L'age-Stehr:

It is good to have serum samples for improved serology, but I think at present we definitely would need to look in mononuclear cells from the peripheral blood for chlamydial DNA, RNA or antigen. Moreover, perhaps we can identify genetic or phenotypic differences in host factor expression like chemokine receptors, cytokines or others. If we would save mononuclear cells, we would have the possibility to look even retrospectively in monocytes or mononuclear cells with improved technology for those factors .

Brade:

I agree with some of the aspects which you mentioned, for example, what are other relevant factors. Please don't mention cytokines. We have already so many people measuring cytokines, not that everyone starts to measure cytokines again: at the DNA level, at the RNA level, at the protein level, inside and outside the cell. The other thing is: what is the information you get with regard to the cytokine network from collecting macrophages?

L'age-Stehr:

I don't mean cytokines quantitatively, but gene expression for cytokine receptors. There may be some differences in persistently infected patients. You know that for example mutations in chemokine receptors are key for cellular HIV uptake. Susceptibility for persistent HIV infection is dependent on these receptors. So why don't we save monocytes or save blood cells?

Brade:
Certainly, the more material you have and the more tests you have, the more information you get. But I think one should also not forget of what is the feasibility of getting the material. To collect serum is certainly the easiest possibility. Many of the studies which we urgently need should not be complicated by making the protocol of collecting materials the limiting factor of a study, as we have heard a couple of minutes ago.

Dunne:
I agree with a lot of the discussion that has been going on. It is a little unclear of how much positive predictive value a single measurement for titers will be, it depends on your cut-off etc. This kind of study is done in the Framingham group, looking at positive predictive value in the future. But perhaps the dynamics of the change in your titer correlating with the dynamics in changing inflammatory response may be more interesting than single values. It kind of gets around the fact that the titers have been measured properly because they all measured the same degree of badness. But at least with time you may see fluctuations correlating with something else and that leading to inflammatory cascade etc. Might that be of more interest over the long haul?

Ziese:
Yes, we did plan this already. What I presented is the first step: that we wanted to confirm or not to confirm the basic theory of there being an association, after controlling for known risk factors. If it is confirmed, we are going to analyze all the serum samples over time. But the first step which I wanted to present here is just to confirm the association which is not yet accepted, as was shown by the discussion today.

4.5
Public health impact of atherosclerosis and *Chlamydia pneumoniae* infections – What do we know and what to expect from future research

J.M. Ossewaarde

Introduction

The association between infectious diseases and atherosclerosis is now well documented [1]. The evidence for involvement of *Chlamydia pneumoniae* in atherogenesis appears to be the strongest. *Chlamydia pneumoniae* infections have been recognized as an independent risk factor for coronary heart disease in a prospective nested case-control study within a cohort of symptom-free elderly men [2]. The number of reports studying the involvement of *Chlamydia pneumoniae* is rapidly rising. This paper summarizes epidemiological data and trends of most prevalent cardiovascular diseases and traditional risk factors in the Netherlands, epidemiological data of *Chlamydia pneumoniae* infections, and of respiratory tract infections as a new risk factor for cardiovascular disease. Combining all this information, we provide suggestions for future research to fill in the gaps in our knowledge of the relationship between *Chlamydia pneumoniae* infections and cardiovascular diseases.

Epidemiology of cardiovascular diseases in the Netherlands

The trends from 1972 to 1993 of the most prevalent cardiovascular diseases and the main risk factors in the Netherlands have been described and reported in 1995 [3]. In 1993, 40 % of all deaths were caused by cardiovascular diseases. Since 1972, cardiovascular diseases mortality decreased, but the total number of hospital admissions of patients older than 65 years for cardiovascular diseases treatment almost doubled (Figure 1). In addition, the mean age at death increased for both males and females. The number of hospital admissions for stroke for males increased from 1972 to 1985 from 135 to 210 per 100,000, followed by a small decrease to 200 per 100,000. The number for females is only slightly smaller. The number of deaths from stroke slightly decreased for males and increased for females, but the age at death is higher than for coronary heart disease, 77.0 y vs. 72.1 y in 1993 for males and 81.7 y vs. 78.8 y in 1993 for females. The number of deaths from abdominal aorta aneurysm in males increased continuously from 1972 to 1993, but not that of females (Figure 2).

Analysis of the three main risk factors showed that the number of male smokers continuously decreased from 90 % in 1958 to 40 % in 1993 (Figure 3). The number of female smokers varied between 35 % and 40 % during this period. Fifteen percent of males older than 45 have hypertension. Four percent of females at age 40 have hypertension, increasing to 18 % at age 60. More than 10 % of males at age 35 have hypercholesterolaemia, increasing to 25 % at age 50. Fifteen percent of females at age 45 have hypercholesterolaemia, increasing to 38 % at age 60. Table 1 shows the prevalence of combinations of these risk factors. A recent analysis in the USA shows, that 25 % of the decrease in coronary heart disease mortality from 1980 to 1990 could be attributed to reduction of these primary risk factors [4]. This summary shows that cardiovascular diseases have a great public health impact and that further research into new risk factors is necessary.

Table 1. Prevalence of combination of risk factors in the general population. Risk factors were: hypercholesterolaemia ($\geq$6.5 mmol/l); hypertension (systolic $\geq$160 mm Hg or diastolic $\geq$95 mm Hg); and smoking of cigarettes.

Number of risk factors	Age	Males	Females
1 risk factor	All	50 %	50 %
2 risk factors	20–29	2 %	<1 %
	30–29	7 %	<1 %
	40–49	12 %	8 %
	50–59	16 %	18 %
3 risk factors	All	1 %	1 %

Epidemiology of *Chlamydia pneumoniae* infections

In a random sample of 1,725 sera collected in 1985 and 1986 from the whole population of the city of Utrecht specific IgG antibodies to *Chlamydia pneumoniae* were determined by enzyme immunoassay [5]. The overall seroprevalence was 56.1 %. After a peak in the age group of 5–10 years, there was an increase in the prevalence of higher titers with age. Since these higher titers are probably associated with recent infections and with the number of reinfections or reactivations, these observations suggest that primary infections occur in childhood and that the number of reinfection and reactivations increases with age. Univariate chi-square analysis was carried out to identify associations with variables from a large questionnaire designed to assess general aspects of health. The questionnaire did not contain specific questions for cardiovascular or respiratory diseases. The analysis revealed a significant correlation between seroprevalence and male gender, ethnic origin from Turkey, use of cardiovascular medication (only in males), use of diuretics, cholesterol level and Quetelet index (only in males from Dutch origin), and smoking of cigarettes (only in females). There was no difference in the percentage of smokers between males and females, but males smoked significantly more cigarettes per day than females (p<0.001). These results suggest that some subpopulations might have a higher risk for *Chlamydia pneumoniae* infections and that *Chlamydia pneumoniae* infections are associated with a number of risk factors for cardiovascular disease. With increasing age, these associations become more pronounced.

Respiratory tract infections as a risk factor for cardiovascular disease

Respiratory tract infections might have immediate effects and long-term effects on cardiovascular diseases. The observed seasonal concurrence of respiratory and cardiovascular mortality suggests an immediate effect of respiratory tract infections on the cardiovascular system [6]. Several pathogenetic explanations have been suggested for this phenomenon, like increased occurrence of thromboembolic processes and enhancement of inflammation in vulnerable sites in atherosclerotic plaques. Thus, respiratory tract infections directly influence or even precipitate the occurrence of cardiovascular incidents. On the other hand, respiratory tract infections also seem to be a risk factor for the progression of atherosclerosis. In a cohort study of almost 20,000 people with a follow-up of 13 years, symptoms of chronic bronchitis were associated with an increased risk for coronary heart disease [7]. This association is confirmed by the observation that antibiotic treatment of acute infections with tetracyclines reduces the risk for coronary heart disease [8]. Thus, respiratory tract infections increase the risk for coronary heart disease and broad-spectrum treatment reduces this increased risk. Respiratory tract infections are also associated with cerebrovascular disease. In a case-control study of 166 consecutive patients with acute cerebrovascular ischaemia and 166 age- and sex-matched non-stroke neurological patient controls, frequent or chronic bronchitis was associated with an increased risk for cerebrovascular disease [9]. Therefore, it is likely that respiratory tract infections induce progression of atherosclerosis.

Association of *Chlamydia pneumoniae* infections and cardiovascular diseases

Chronic and recurrent *Chlamydia pneumoniae* infections are not only associated with an increased risk for coronary heart diseases [1], but also with a number of risk factors. Primary reduction of traditional risk factors explains only 25 % of the decline in coronary heart disease mortality in the USA, while technical treatment improvements and secondary prevention explained 72 % [4]. Therefore, there is ample room for improvement in primary prevention strategies. To design these strategies, more information is needed on the association of *Chlamydia pneumoniae* infections with other risk factors for cardiovascular diseases. However, interactions between risk factors are complex, statistically as well as biologically. Only a few studies have addressed the association of *Chlamydia pneumoniae* infections with other risk factors for coronary heart diseases. In a study of 415 males studied two times with an interval of three years subjects with chronic infection with *Chlamydia pneumoniae* defined by persistence of IgG and IgA antibodies were compared with subjects that were antibody negative on both occasions [10]. An atherogenic lipid profile characterized by an increase in total cholesterol and a decrease in HDL cholesterol was associated with chronic *Chlamydia pneumoniae* infections. Smoking of cigarettes is associated with an increased risk for respiratory tract infections [11]. Although not yet proven, it is likely that *Chlamydia pneumoniae* infections are not different from viral infections in this respect. Thus, *Chlamydia pneumoniae* infections can be a confounder in the relation between smoking of cigarettes and cardiovascular diseases [12]. Smoking of cigarettes was also associated with *Chlamydia pneumoniae* infections in the Finnish Twin Cohort study [13]. The definition of confounding is a distortion of an exposure–outcome association brought about by the association of another factor with both outcome and exposure (Figure 4). *Chlamydia pneumoniae* infections can be considered as a confounding factor in the relationship between smoking of cigarettes and cardiovascular diseases (Figure 5) and between an atherogenic lipid profile and cardiovascular diseases (Figure 6). The exact role of *Chlamydia pneumoniae* infections in these relationships is unknown. A causal relationship of *Chlamydia pneumoniae* infections and cardiovascular diseases has not been proven yet. Although the question of absolute proof of an infectious cause of cardiovascular diseases is irrelevant, more data would be helpful to further enhance our understanding and to find answers for causal criteria like Elwood's comprehensive scheme for the assessment of causation [14]. Especially an estimate of the preventable fraction of cardiovascular diseases attributed to *Chlamydia pneumoniae* infections is needed to assess the cost–benefit of preventive measures like antibiotic treatment and vaccines. Carefully designed trials might provide some answers.

Public health consequences

Information on demographic characteristics of individuals with respiratory infections and cardiovascular diseases permits identification of high-risk groups, while information on specific infections and risk factors may provide possible clues of etiologic agents or modes of spread. Before deciding to take primary or secondary preventive measures, available evidence should be critically assessed. Standard guidelines for this procedure do not exist for any type of disease, including chronic infectious diseases. However, generally evidence is categorized in one of four hierarchy levels: 1) randomized trials; 2) cohort or case-control studies; 3) comparative studies; 4) case reports, descriptive studies, and professional experience. To implement measures that are more drastic, solid evidence of the first level is needed. Surveillance data combined with epidemiologic investigations might suggest early prevention recommendations and evaluate effectiveness of interventions. Finally, public health measures will also be based on technical progress, cost–benefit analysis, and political decisions.

Conclusions

From a public health point of view, the association between *Chlamydia pneumoniae* infections and cardiovascular diseases is of great importance. To assess the need for measures on a (sub)population level, more information is needed on the interaction between *Chlamydia pneumoniae* infections and risk factors for cardiovascular diseases as well as the risk for cardiovascular disease attributable to *Chlamydia pneumoniae* infections.

Acknowledgments

The author thanks Prof. D. Kromhout and Dr. T.G. Kimman for their constructive comments during the preparation of the manuscript.

References

1. Danesh J, Collins R, Peto R (1997) Chronic infections and coronary heart disease: is there a link? Lancet 350: 430–436
2. Ossewaarde JM, Feskens EJM, De Vries A, Vallinga CE, Kromhout D (1998) *Chlamydia pneumoniae* is a risk factor for coronary heart disease in symptom free elderly men, but *Helicobacter pylori* and cytomegalovirus are not. Epidemiol Infect 120: 93–99
3. Reitsma JB (1995) Hart – en vaatziekten in Nederland 1995. Nederlandse Hartstichting, Den Haag
4. Hunink MGM, Goldman L, Tosteson ANA, Mittleman MA, Goldman PA, Williams LW, Tsevat J, Weinstein MC (1997) The recent decline in mortality from coronary heart disease, 1980–1990. The effect of secular trends in risk factors and treatment. JAMA 277: 535–542
5. Ossewaarde JM, Van Steenbergen JE, Van der Meijden-Kuypers HL, Gorissen WHM (1995) Seroepidemiology of *Chlamydia pneumoniae* infections in the city of Utrecht, The Netherlands. Atherosclerosis 115 (Suppl.): S122
6. Crombie DL, Fleming DM, Cross KW, Lancashire RJ (1995) Concurrence of monthly variations of mortality related to underlying cause in Europe. J Epidemiol Community Health 49: 373–378
7. Jousilahti P, Vartiainen E, Tuomilehto J, Puska P (1996) Symptoms of chronic bronchitis and the risk of coronary disease. Lancet 348: 567–572
8. Meier CR, Derby LE, Jick SS, Vasilakis C, Jick H (1999) Antibiotics and risk of subsequent first-time acute myocardial infarction. JAMA 281: 427–431
9. Grau AJ, Buggle F, Ziegler C, Schwarz W, Meuser J, Tasman AJ, Buhler A, Benesch C, Becher H, Hacke W (1997) Association between acute cerebrovascular ischemia and chronic and recurrent infection. Stroke 28: 1724–1729
10. Laurila A, Bloigu A, Näyhä S, Hassi J, Leinonen M, Saikku P (1997) Chronic *Chlamydia pneumoniae* infection is associated with a serum lipid profile known to be a risk factor for atherosclerosis. Arterioscler Thromb Vasc Biol 17: 2910–2913
11. Cohen S, Tyrrell DAJ, Russell MAH, Jarvis MJ, Smith AP (1993) Smoking, alcohol consumption, and susceptibility to the common cold. Am J Publ Health 83: 1277–1283
12. Hahn DL, Golubjatnikov R (1992) Smoking is a potential confounder of the *Chlamydia pneumoniae* coronary artery disease association. Arterioscl Thromb 12: 945–947
13. Von Hertzen L, Surcel HM, Kaprio J, Koskenvuo M, Bloigu A, Leinonen M, Saikku P (1998) Immune responses to *Chlamydia pneumoniae* in twins in relation to gender and smoking. J Med Microbiol 47: 441–446
14. Elwood JM (1998) Critical appraisal of epidemiological studies and clinical trials. Oxford University Press, Oxford, Second edition

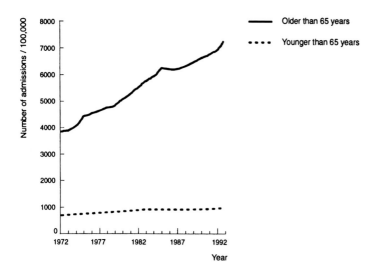

Figure 1. Number of hospital admissions for treatment of cardiovascular diseases per 100,000 of the total population.

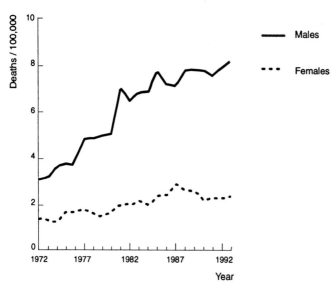

Figure 2. Number of deaths due to abdominal aortic aneurysms per 100,000 of the total population.

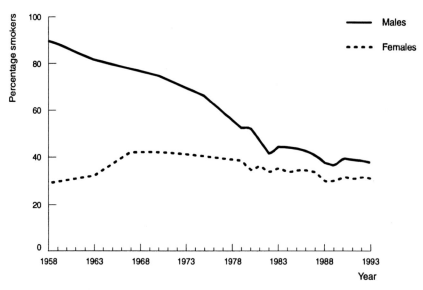

Figure 3. Trend of percentage of smokers in the general population.

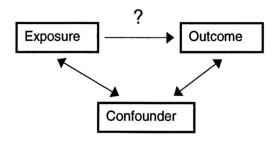

Figure 4. Theoretical graphical representation of possible associations between a confounder and both the exposure and the outcome.

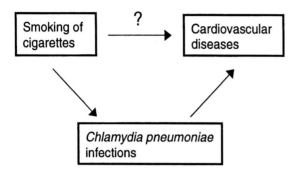

Figure 5. Theoretical graphical representation of associations between *Chlamydia pneumoniae* infections, smoking of cigarettes and cardiovascular diseases. Is the action of smoking of cigarettes directly responsible for the occurrence of cardiovascular diseases or via *Chlamydia pneumoniae* infections?

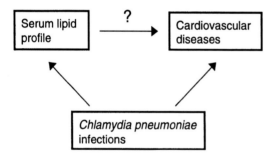

Figure 6. Theoretical graphical representation of associations between *Chlamydia pneumoniae* infections, an atherogenic lipid profile and cardiovascular diseases. Is an atherogenic lipid profile a risk factor for cardiovascular diseases or is an atherogenic lipid profile a result of the action of *Chlamydia pneumoniae* infections?

Discussion

Stille:

I think infectious diseases and trauma should not be compared. The epidemiology in both is too different. The role risk factors play in trauma is different from that in a chronic inflammatory infectious disease, it is difficult to compare. The risk factor concept in for instance car accidents has a totally different position from that in tuberculosis.

Ossewaarde:

You are completely right. But on the other hand maybe it is true that once you have had a chlamydial infection you have some kind of sensibilization of the vascular wall and atherosclerosis might develop. Just as when you have had a head trauma and a disturbed equilibrium, later on when something else happens you break your hip. The interaction of all those risk factors involved in atherosclerosis is very complicated.

Stille:

Are the risk factors really so complicated? With a simple chronic disease you do not need risk factors primarily, you have secondary risk factors which are very important, but primarily you have a chronic smoldering infection like syphilis.

Ossewaarde:

In syphilis you have just one agent, in atherosclerosis many agents might be involved. I have mentioned dental infections in which there are at least two different bacteria involved, and cytomegalovirus. Helicobacter is involved, maybe herpes simplex virus, *C. pneumoniae*, and maybe other chlamydia-like microorganisms we don't know about at this moment. It is a whole group of organisms and also a whole group of infections because three studies I showed on recurrent respiratory tract infections show that respiratory tract infections are risk factors for cardiovascular disease on a long term, not on a short term within a couple of days or one week. That is different.

Byrne:

It may even become more fundamental than that. I think everyone would agree with me, we have an inflammatory disease and are wrestling with the question: do one or more infectious agents contribute to that inflammation? Or are risk factors that don't involve infections sufficient? I think that is sort of where we are at, and that is where the room is quite divided right down the middle now.

Chapter 5
Final Discussion: Pro and Contra the Role of *Chlamydia pneumoniae* in Chronic Diseases

Burger:
Prof. Stille suggested a short talk by Dr. May from Munich in addition to the agenda in order to demonstrate that also in Germany randomized decent studies can be performed.

May:
I would like to shortly present our randomized prospective study from Munich which deals with the therapy of macrolides for patients suffering from coronary artery disease. The question we ask is: Does a four-week therapy with roxithromycin lower the rate of restenosis in patients undergoing coronary stent implantation? As you know, the development of restenosis after coronary stent implantation remains to be a major problem in the field of cardiology, and the reason for the development of restenosis is yet unknown.

The inclusion criterion for patients is a successful coronary stent implantation, exclusion criteria are contraindications against roxithromycin. The major endpoint is the rate of restenosis after six months and a secondary endpoint is the combined clinical endpoint of death, myocardial infarction or the need for coronary revascularization by PTCA or coronary bypass operation. We further try to answer some additional questions: Is there a relationship between Chlamydia or CMV titers and the rate of restenosis after a coronary stent implantation, and does a relationship exist between inflammatory parameters, infectious parameters and the rate of restenosis?

The study protocol is quite easy. Patients that undergo coronary stent implantation are randomized for either placebo or roxithromycin 300 mg a day for four weeks, and they all undergo reangiography after a period of 6 months. We also determine some laboratory parameters at two timepoints: the time of the intervention and the time of re-coronary angiography after six months. As inflammatory markers we choose C-reactive protein and interleukin-6, and as infectious markers we determine the titers of *C. pneumoniae* and CMV. We try to study Chlamydiae in circulating monocytes. Given that you have a rate of restenosis in the placebo group of 28 % after six months, our statistics department calculated that you can show at least a 30 % reduction of the rate of restenosis significantly with the power of 80 % if you have about 1,000 patients (500 patients per group). At this timepoint we have included 800 patients and are planning to finish the study around the middle of the year. I am sorry to only be able to present the design of the study, since we do not have the data available yet.

Burger:

Thank you, Dr. May. After these invited contributions we come to the general discussion of this meeting and have a number of questions listed in program:

- pro and contra relevant role of *C. pneumoniae* infections in pathogenesis of chronic diseases
- deficits and goals in clinical and epidemiological research
- critical points in study designs
- development of better diagnostic tools
- primary and secondary prevention of infection
- impact on public health and future goals

This may be a somewhat difficult discussion because we might want to avoid that the saying of the famous Bavarian humorist Karl Valentin applies to us who once said, "everything has been said but not yet by everybody". We ought to concentrate on the topics above and perhaps include some new arguments in this discussion instead of repeating arguments which were made already in the course of the last two days.

Straube:

Actually our topic should be chronic chlamydial infection, and we should not only talk about coronary heart disease but also about other chlamydial infective entities. There is a need for several studies in the pathogenesis of coronary heart disease according to what we have heard from the Robert Koch-Institut and from Frankfurt. We should look for good laboratories which could provide valid diagnostic methods to improve the studies.

Ossewaarde:

I have a question for Dr. Bhakdi on his new hypothesis on LDL and atherosclerosis. If I understand it correctly, when the LDL moves to the subendothelial space, it becomes modified and is then atherogenic and removed by monocytes/macrophages?

Bhakdi:

Yes, HDL plays the important role of obtaining the cholesterol from the foam cells, that is why HDL is antiatherogenic. The LDL/HDL quotient is important.

Ossewaarde:

But if I hypothetically removed monocytes/macrophages, then the lesion would aggregate?

Bhakdi:

This experiment would be of great interest. But we ourselves cannot do it.

Ossewaarde:

A couple of weeks ago, there was a paper in *Nature* in which they used knockout mice for monocyte receptors. There were no monocytes in the lesions and the lesions were not enhanced, they did not occur. So without monocytes there were no lesions but a lot of LDL.

Bhakdi:

This tells you that the role of the monocyte is indeed central. There are two effectors: complement and monocytes. The prediction would be, if you remove any one of these, you will improve the outcome. This has been shown in the paper you cite. We show that by knocking out complement you also get protection. Vice versa, if you infuse activated macrophages in the lesion, the lesion gets worse. And it doesn't matter where the infection is, it doesn't have to be in the vascular system, it can be anywhere. In fact, it doesn't have to be an infection at all.

Ossewaarde:

In your model, how do you see the complications of atherosclerotic disease? Plaque instability?

Bhakdi:

We do not know. The progression of the lesion is something we do not touch on. We are seeing that there are three parts: the initiation, the progression and the complications. I don't believe that there are three different diseases, but we are restricting ourselves to the initiation stage.

Maass:

There are still many open questions. The most important ones refer to the biological and to the clinical relevance of *C. pneumoniae* in the pathogenesis of chronic vascular infections. We should remember that findings are still contradictory and that there is no scientific proof that *C. pneumoniae* contributes to atherosclerosis. In addition, it is important to improve the diagnostic assays for *C. pneumoniae* infections, not only in regard to vascular diseases but also in regard to respiratory diseases. We are lacking a standardized clinically evaluated diagnostic assay for *C. pneumoniae* infections. It is an important objective to develop a method that is rapid (because the patients are in need of treatment), reliable and able to detect viable infective microorganisms. With such a method, some of the problems discussed here may be solved. Another important step are common efforts, as the one Jens Boman has initiated for the external evaluation of PCR methods in different laboratories, a prerequisite to improve the diagnosis of *C. pneumoniae* and to make data more comparable between the laboratories.

Stratton:

We were arguing whether the chicken or the egg comes first. Why do we need to have it either/or? Jens Boman has done a very nice paper showing that peripheral blood mononuclear cells have got *C. pneumoniae* in them. Other investigators have, at least to me, shown that this is probably a metabolizing organism or supposedly just some DNA that is hanging around. If you got peripheral blood mononuclear cells that are infected with Chlamydia, then you have inflammation. You can define inflammation with two characteristics, white cell recruitment and angiogenesis, and we have two of the favored substrates of Chlamydia. If the peripheral blood mononuclear cells are infected and they go to the inflamed area (whether it is in the brain or in the coronary or somewhere else), why can't you get a chronic chlamydial secondary infection that then becomes what we call multiple sclerosis or coronary artery disease or something else? For example, your LPS theory might be exactly correct for the etiology of atherosclerosis, but it is the chronically infected monocytes that prolong it.

Byrne:
Just a comment on the point Dr. Maass made which relates to optimizing conditions to repeat the types of studies that have been done. We really do need that – more laboratories and more people – and more investigations that are competently done. But in terms of getting at the issue, what more would this audience like to see in terms of either defining whether Chlamydia are present differently or doing additional experiments to show causality or developing new animal models? I would like to know, is there something really unique or something new that has not been done competently by somebody, at least once, oftentimes more than once? Or whether what we need to do is have verification of things that have been done?

Maass:
It is important that some publications stated that most of the specimens from vascular tissue were negative by PCR. The differences in the detection rates were clearly dependent on the method used. I think the methodology has first to be evaluated before we start further investigations. A noteworthy point that already has become clear in the last four years is that the tiny vascular samples obtained from rotational catheter ablation procedures during coronary angiography are not useful to detect *C. pneumoniae*, as the groups using those samples find no or only very few positives.

Byrne:
I wonder if the answer to that question might at least in part be completed if we develop some sort of reference laboratory system. Maybe that is really what we need, rather than have any lab who wants to analyze Chlamydia do it, and do it by methods that may or may not be appropriate. To have some subset of central laboratories that should be, at least initially, screened for their competence, this would help a lot in terms of getting at that issue.

Bauriedel:
Two short comments to the current discussion: when we used immunohistochemistry, we also were able to find the same strong difference between the two patient groups (stable angina and unstable angina) when looking at the chlamydial heat-shock protein 60. So I think these are valid data.

My second point: Dr. May, what makes you so sure that you have looked at the right target population when you study restenosis? What is your evidence when you treat these people with a macrolide?

May:
There is no evidence right now but it works. That is why we are performing this study. The problem of restenosis is not solved right now. We only know that there is a mechanical injury that induces restenosis and some people, about 30 or 40, develop a restenosis. If these people develop a restenosis, the chance to develop another restenosis is very high in these patients. There are some links that show that there must be a special cause for the development of restenosis. We have heard enough data for the last two days showing that *C. pneumoniae* or CMV may trigger the development of restenosis as well as atherosclerosis.

Stille:
I have to defend the Munich group. They did not discuss it, they really did the treatment. On the other hand, the rate of restenosis in stents with up to 40 % is absolutely unacceptable for a medical treatment. Also in dilatation the rate of restenosis is high, therefore they implant the stent. If you start from the condition there, if you dilate tuberculous endarteritis, a disease which is very rare in Germany, you will get an immediate local reactivation. Probably you have the same with Chlamydia. There is a high percentage of complication, and we can show that if we reduce the complication, we are on the right track and can show it in a short time.

Bhakdi:
You are considering that infections may promote or accelerate the lesions. There is nothing against that, except that one has to try to find out what is the weight of these factors. Studies clearly show that you can get very dramatic lesion regression without antibiotics. Therefore infections cannot play the major role.
May I ask Dr. May, are your patients all getting statins?

May:
Not all of them.

Bhakdi:
Why not? How many percent are getting statins? Because that of course is evidence-based medicine. We know that this treatment is indicated for your patient group. Are you treating patients without statins, with only one antibiotic?

Stille:
No, the effect of statins is poor. Statins do not work in the beginning, they work after two years. When you look to the 4S study ("Scandinavian Simvastatin Survival Study") and all these classical studies, you see a difference after two years. Statins are long-term treatment agents, while antibiotics are short-term treatment agents.

Bhakdi:
As far as I know, there are hard data to say that your patients are all on the list for statins. If you don't give them statins, you are withholding therapy. In the *New England Journal of Medicine* of the 5th of November 1998, read the next to the last paragraph in the LIPID Study article: only 10 % of patients in Europe who should receive statins are being treated. If evidence-based medicine says, this is clear, then it should be followed. If you were doing animal experiments, I would not mind, but we are looking at thousands of patients.

Byrne:
On the one hand, you are following "Occams Razor" very nicely and you are not complicating the situation, because you feel like you don't have to, which is what William of Occam would have advised. But on the other hand, I think we have a complicated situation. I don't think it is an either/or, one-answer situation. You are trying to make it out to be that way, so that you are as impatient in your view as most chlamydia-promoting individuals would be in their view with possibly less data. There are a lot of data on the statins, and certainly lipid-lowering drugs are important, but it is not exclusive of other things.

Stille:
Nobody says that.

Bauriedel:
We clearly have to differentiate between different forms of atherosclerosis. We have early stages, advanced lesions and restenosis. I am very thankful that in our study we used stenting, since we know very well that restenosis in stent is a different type from chronic atherosclerosis. Therefore I cannot agree with Dr. Stille on that. Intimal hyperplasia is a high cellularity of viable smooth muscle cells. This is totally different from all these other stages of atherosclerosis we have already discussed, and I am very skeptic that you will have any results in that, since there is no clear evidence for that. There is one study in *Circulation* from Prof. Strauer's group from Düsseldorf who could show no association between serologic parameters and restenosis. In the paper from Steve Epsteins group, there is the hypothesis of an antiapoptotic virus-induced activity in the plaques leading to increased cellularity. But these parameters and determinants have not yet been isolated and detected in the plaques directly.

Brade:
To start with the word of our former chancellor Helmut Kohl, "the caravan is moving on, no matter what we are discussing here". That is very clear from this meeting and from other meetings where most of the people met in this or that mixture. The way it is going on, there is no chance anymore to say that these studies, these antibiotic trials will not be done. The keypoint of further antibiotic studies will be: is there a positive effect or not?

The second thing is, we need better research in Chlamydia. In Germany no one better than me can say this. In this audience I think in Germany I am the one who has been working longest on Chlamydia, for more than 25 years. I have always had problems in convincing people that we need basic research. For me it was the LPS – as you all know I've been working all the time on this single molecule – and I was told no more than five or six years ago by reviewers in Germany that our projects on the chlamydial LPS were academic playing and that this was not necessary. If I wanted to do something relevant, I should work on proteins. I said, ok, I will do my work with the resources which I have available. I could give you many more examples. Within the Chlamydia society – and here are long-lasting members present who could confirm this – there is so much more to do than to improve a PCR protocol or a serological assay.

If in a couple of years it turned out that a certain fraction of atherosclerotic patients definitely improved from an antibiotic treatment, I think it is clear to us that that will not be long-lasting because we don't have the appropriate antibiotics. Today pharmaceutical companies should already think about developing new antibiotics instead of modifying them. Antibiotics have been developed 50–60 years ago, and really nothing new came out because they always modified antibiotics to make them fit better this or that microorganism. Someone will come up with a completely new concept of developing antibiotics, and I can tell you from my own work, I have offered to look for glycosol transferase inhibitors to interfere at a completely different pathway.

The question of vaccination also came up. In case antibiotic treatment is not feasible because we do not have the proper compounds to treat patients, and if atherosclerosis starts at 15 years (as I have learned today), or let us say at 30, when you have two additional risk factors, you start with antibiotic prevention. Is anyone in this room willing to take macrolides for 30, 40 years? Certainly not. So with vaccination I see another problem. We have learned from much of the work being done in the US: half the Chlamydia society was sponsored by the NIH, claiming that they were developing a vaccine against trachoma. That work has been going on for a long time and the trachoma vaccine will not come.

We should not forget we are at the Robert Koch-Institut, we will certainly be getting an opinion by the Robert Koch-Institut about what is relevant for Germany or perhaps relevant in Europe with regard to chlamydial diseases. If we start to improve research on Chlamydia, I would propose we should start at the early beginnings. First I would like to see someone determine what the signals are in the differentiation between EBs and RBs. If we understood what happens at the molecular level, maybe an antibiotic treatment would be much easier if we could get all the resting elementary bodies or all the silent bodies. Mulder described the silent bodies but nobody knows what they actually are. If you had all Chlamydia in a replicative stage, maybe then antibiotic treatment would be key. I could give you a whole list of "most important" things which should first be studied before at the end of this line we are improving the microimmunofluorescence assay or a PCR protocol or a culture protocol, as long as we have not understood why under natural conditions we cannot infect tissue culture cells. If you are looking to these systems in which we are multiplying a microorganism which is involved in such complicated diseases like reactive arthritis or atherosclerosis, we don't understand why these microbes are not growing in tissue culture cells. There is so much to do and I would be happy if this meeting helps to raise funds. We have been fighting for a long time. If we get money for this research, then it is worth that we are fighting again and again.

Maass:

There is no alternative to further research, of course. It is important to work with this organism very sincerely and in experienced laboratories. We need reference laboratories to eliminate the differences between the diagnostic tests. Not everybody should have to establish his own in-house *C. pneumoniae* serology and PCR. With specialized laboratories, the diagnostic quality will improve. On the basis of the occurrence of viable bacteria in plaques, we have started antibiotic treatment trials. We need those trials, but we do not want everybody with a heart problem to take antibiotics, and this may well be a result of the current discussions. In the lay press there are already headlines like: "myocardial infarction can be treated with antibiotics". In fact, it cannot. But we need trials to show whether antibiotics are effective or not. Even if the pathogenetic idea of chlamydial involvement is correct, this does not necessarily result in a well-treatable condition. Persistent chlamydial infection can be expected to be a serious challenge of the current conception of antimicrobial treatment. There is no alternative to the extension of the research activities on Chlamydiae and atherosclerosis.

Christiansen:

I totally agree with Dr. Brade that a lot more research should be done on Chlamydia. I hope that with this meeting which I really have enjoyed we can initiate some more collaboration with everybody who is doing clinical trials, molecular biology, LPS research and so on. Collaboration may be under this new EU 5th program, where one of the prerequisites is the multitude of things that should be studied, in order not to have too many programs. I recommend this as one of the possibilities to apply for.

We should focus on whether this is a clonal lineage of a bug or whether there are different lineages. We should study why do they have families of genes with a very limited genome, when are they using what kind of turn-on of genes. Not only the omp2 and 3 and the histone-like proteins later in the life cycle, but also other things that we haven't even thought of yet. By going into Rick Stephens' database with the *C. pneumoniae* genome and comparing it to the *C. trachomatis* genome, it is possible to find ways to look for specific things that we have not even thought of yet. Without doing that, we can waste a lot of time just looking for things that have been partly studied without really confirmative analysis.

I think we should look for risk factors. Probably serology may not be very useful because you look at what is always there on the surface. But maybe some of the genes that are turned on under specific conditions will create a possibility to look for risk factors. Many things should be done but I think they should be standardized better. It shouldn't happen that one group can come up with 100 % of something and others with 0 %, if this has not been done by tests that have been approved of to be of similar efficacy. There is a lot of standardization to do and I hope that this also could come out of this meeting.

Dr. Brade, I can tell you that my first student actually just started a new company in Denmark with about 25 million German Marks for making new antibiotic treatment tests by a totally new concept, where they have a patent on PNA, the protein like DNA that they have targeted in a way so they can go into bacteria and in that way inhibit specific necessary genes when they are active.

May:
Dr. Bhakdi, of course we are treating patients with statins and the aim of the LDL level is below 110–120 in our clinic. It is still a point of discussion if you have to treat any patient with statins after stent implantation or with coronary artery disease.

Dr. Bauriedel, of course I think atherosclerosis and restenosis are different diseases but they both depend on inflammatory triggers, and it is well known that restenosis is induced by inflammatory triggers peri- and postinterventionally and, for example, in knock-out mice suffering from the deficiency of adhesion molecules on monocytes. When monocytes cannot migrate into the inflammatory tissue, restenosis is totally absent in these mice. Therefore a trigger such as *C. pneumoniae* that induces and activates monocytes and granulocytes may have an effect on the development of restenosis, at least in my opinion.

Stille:
This is a discussion pro and contra. Within the last minutes the discussion contra has had a stronger position. I stand for the position pro and I want to stress that the explanation of atherosclerosis as chronic chlamydial infection is much better than the existing theories where atherosclerosis is evaluated as chronic intoxication or chronic metabolic disease due to some errors in metabolism of cholesterol. We ought to stress far more what is to be done, what do we expect from the Robert Koch-Institut, our host, what do we expect from the German government? The real money is spent by the *Forschungsministerium*. What do we expect from the German and also the international medical community? I am sure that certain questions cannot be solved in Germany, certain questions need a closed society. For instance, long-term epidemiological studies should be made in countries like Iceland where you have a good medical system and a defined and stable population. It cannot be done in Berlin where people stay for five years and then disappear.

On the other hand, I want to stress to not waste your time on investigations on pathogenesis. Take for example a classical disease like tuberculosis. We know the course of tuberculosis, we know risk factors, we have a perfect treatment, but we do not need to know everything concerning the pathogenesis of tuberculosis. It takes decades, maybe centuries, until in the end you really understand the complete pathogenesis of a disease, if you understand it at all. In my opinion – I just want to put this forward and leave it hanging in the air –, are we justified in being so obstructive against treatment? We have to ask, from what point onward is it unethical to withhold from a patient a treatment with antibiotics? The 38-year-old patient and coronary infarction without risk factors, these patients are not uncommon, or the patients with young stroke shortly after respiratory infection or patients with multiple sclerosis. There is no real established treatment of multiple sclerosis, every therapy existing has an efficiency of only around 20 %. What shall we do with a patient with rapidly progressive multiple sclerosis? In a case of a non-treatable disease it is justified to "clutch at any straw", so interventional treatment is justified already now. I am strictly against preventive treatment. Nobody should go and treat all 40-year-old persons with antibiotics without any sign of atherosclerosis. This would be the wrong way for the time being. But interventional therapy and studies and interventional treatment groups with protocols are already justified at the moment. The treatment for all conventional widespread diseases was not detected in large-scale randomized studies, it was direct observational treatment. If a principle works, you will find it even in an open study.

Maass:

Gunna Christiansen has mentioned the research network of the 5th EC research plan. We should use this workshop here in Berlin at the Robert Koch-Institut to initiate such a network on chlamydial research. There are so many potential partners from Europe here who could improve their co-operation substantially. There are also many partners from the United States who also could co-operate. In the EC plan there are many possibilities to combine basic with applied research. It clearly meets the objectives of the 5th EC research plan to improve our knowledge on the biology of *C. pneumoniae* and *C. trachomatis*, perhaps also on the biology of *C. psittaci*, and to develop pertinent diagnostic and therapeutic applications.

Burger:

Perhaps I may take the privilege of the moderator to make a few closing remarks, particularly as someone not directly involved in the Chlamydia work who may have a little more distance.

In retrospect, I realize that this meeting was quite informative and that it was justified to bring the experts together and to hear the contributions of the various speakers here in this discussion. Particularly in the sometimes rather critical discussions the speakers not only presented an overview of the different areas of research, but also did not omit the aspects which are unclear and require clarification, and they clearly emphasized these controversial topics. I think this is helpful in a period where plans are made about the future course.

Sometimes conflicting opinions became quite obvious, and sometimes not only the opinions or the interpretations were different but also the results. A number of principal questions remain which require an answer, not only whether Chlamydia causes diseases or not, or which diseases; the pathomechanisms remain to be defined, the real cause of the disease. My impression is that a number of unanswered, rather basic questions require immediate action, for instance persistence or the detection of the organism *in situ*, also *in vitro*. The relevance of serology and of other methods like PCR was also questioned. Validations are required and several times a need for standards was mentioned. There are well-established systems to define reference standards which prove to be quite helpful in the field of infectious agents, for instance hepatitis. Also, basic problems like isolation or culture *in vitro*, immunohistology and the relevance of the data from these studies probably need more standardization or evaluation.

In other words, in many areas a solid basic platform has to be at least improved, perhaps sometimes even established for really informative and viable conclusions. A wide spectrum of diseases was discussed here, in addition to the major topic atherosclerosis other diseases like asthma and diseases of the central nervous system, including multiple sclerosis or Alzheimer. A few of you were obviously uncomfortable that the spectrum of diseases was a little too broad. You mentioned that yesterday quite clearly. Chlamydia obviously is a multidisciplinary object and requires cooperation from epidemiologists, clinicians or microbiologists, across the borders of the various specialties.

As you know, this meeting was also envisaged as a means for the Robert Koch-Institut to find its position regarding this infectious agent and to define the need where the Robert Koch-Institut as central institution in the German health system might contribute to analysis and perhaps also to progress. Before a rapid and maybe premature statement might be given right now, we here at the institute should first digest this meeting properly and perhaps have some internal additional discussion before reaching a conclusion. Some of the first ideas or proposals were clearly raised today in this discussion.

I wish to cordially thank the persons organizing this meeting, particularly Frau Dr. L'age-Stehr, but also the others involved in the background.

Acknowledgements

For valuable assistance in organizing the workshop we cordially thank K. Bergemann, S. Berger, A. Brauer, H. Emmel, D. Naumann, J.-W. Sim-Brandenburg and M. Urban-Schriefer.

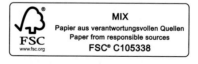

Printed by Books on Demand, Germany